Measuring Medical Education

The Tests and Test Procedures of the

National Board of Medical Examiners

Measuring Medical Education

The Tests and Test Procedures of the National Board of Medical Examiners

John P. Hubbard, M.D.

President, National Board of Medical Examiners
Professor Emeritus, University of Pennsylvania School of Medicine

with a chapter by
Charles F. Schumacher, Ph.D.
Associate Director, National Board of Medical Examiners

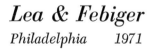

Lea & Febiger
Philadelphia   1971

ISBN 0-8121-0365-3

Library of Congress Catalog Card Number 77–170736

Published in Great Britain by Henry Kimpton Publishers, London

Printed in the United States of America

To my wife, Dorothy, whose understanding and patience are among the manifestations of her true affection.

Preface

This volume deals with the ways in which the National Board of Medical Examiners creates, scores, analyzes and reports objective examinations that provide valid and reliable measurements of the knowledge and clinical competence of medical students, physicians in training and physicians in practice. The measurements of individuals, who are the product of the educational system, may be analyzed and studied collectively for classes of students and groups of physicians at varying points of development, thereby yielding objective assessments of the effectiveness of the educational system. Evaluation of the product thus provides evaluation of the process.

We do not wish to imply that objective measurements obtained by examinations are necessarily the most appropriate or best methods of evaluating medical students or medical education. The continuous assessment of individual students by their own faculties has advantages that cannot be superseded by formal, sporadic extramural examinations, no matter how good the latter may be. At the institutional level, on-site surveys, studies of educational facilities, and face-to-face interviews with faculty and students, as conducted by visiting teams from the American Medical Association, the Association of American Medical Colleges, the specialty boards and societies, have become well established as the mechanisms for approval of medical schools and graduate training programs.

Objective measurements of medical knowledge and competence, as described in the following chapters, have, however, introduced a new and useful dimension of the educational system. With due recognition of the variability in the raw material of medical education, that is, the students as they enter medical school, their medical knowledge and competence as measured at intervals along the educational path provide assessments, limited though they may be, of the educational process.

These assessments and the methods of obtaining them as described in the following chapters are the outgrowth of twenty years of experience in the application of the science of educational measurement to the science of medicine. This experience began in 1950 when the National Board of Medical Examiners, with the assistance of the Educational Testing Service, undertook to introduce multiple-choice testing methods. We remain deeply grateful for the cooperation of the ETS during the years 1951 to 1955 and for their help in establishing the psychometric principles which characterize our examinations today.

In 1956, the working relationship with the ETS was discontinued when the National Board brought psychometric competence into its own organization with the appointment of William V. Clemans, Ph.D., to the full-time staff. This created one of the special features of the National Board: individuals with training and experience in educational measurement working together in a close team relationship with those of the staff who have had experience in medical education as students and as faculty members. Doctor Clemans, who left the staff of the National Board of Medical Examiners in 1961 for a position with Science Research Associates, deserves lasting thanks for his contribution to the development of the Board's examination system and for having been coauthor of *Multiple-Choice Examinations in Medicine,* a small volume which has served as a guide for examiner and examinee both at home and abroad.

As the demands on the services of the National Board have grown, so too has the staff, but always endeavoring to maintain a balance between those with backgrounds in medicine and medical education and those with backgrounds in psychometrics. Although all deserve recognition for their roles in the procedures and accomplishments described in the following pages, special recognition is due to the two senior Associate Directors: Edithe J. Levit, M.D., and Charles F. Schumacher, Ph.D.

Doctor Levit's creative imagination, tireless energy and persuasive leadership are responsible for many of the innovative developments that have become regular features of the Board's examinations. Her influence was first apparent in the introduction of the objective measurements of clinical competence that have characterized the Board's Part III examinations for ten years, that have been adopted by American specialty boards, and that have led to the research and development of the computerized system of evaluating clinical competence described in Chapter 12. Her pioneering work with the American Board of Neurological Surgery and the Association of Neurological Surgeons (Chapter 9) has demonstrated ways in which sophisticated examination procedures can be used as guides to learning for physicians in training at the graduate level. At the undergraduate medical-school level, she developed and popularized the "Minitest" (Chapter 9) as a sequential evaluation of the learning process.

Doctor Schumacher, who came to the National Board of Medical Examiners from the Research Division of the Association of American Medical Colleges, succeeded Doctor Clemans in bringing to the Board the needed strength in the field of educational measurement. During a period of rapid expansion, his unswerving adherence to the principles of psychometrics coupled with an innate sense of research have kept progress tempered with realism. His chapter on scoring and analysis (Chapter 6) is his most directly recognizable contribution to this volume, but his hand is also to be seen in all of the chapters and, more especially, in the work that makes them possible.

Other members of the professional staff deserve recognition for their roles in the activities of the Board which are the substance of this volume. William B. Kennedy, M.D., formerly Associate Dean at the University of Pennsylvania School of Medicine, has had special responsibility for the Board's examinations in the basic medical sciences and the clinical sciences (Parts I and II) and for many of the examinations derived from the Board's pool of tested and standardized examination material (Chapter 8). Alfred R. Stumpe, M.D., was Chief of the Division of Graduate Medical Education for the United States Air Force before he joined the staff of the National Board. He is, therefore, exceptionally well qualified for his present increasing responsibilities for examination programs for specialty boards and specialty societies. Paul R. Kelley, Jr., Ph.D., the number two man on the psychometric team, shares with Doctor Schumacher the credit for solid reliable adherence to basic principles and the achievement of the staff in keeping up with the demands for increasing services. Bryce Templeton, M.D., with a background as Assistant Professor of Psychiatry at the University of Pittsburgh and with a year of study in research in medical education at the University of Illinois, brings to the staff his interest in the expanding influence of behavioral science in medical education and his zest for new and better ways of assessing some of the more elusive but nonetheless essential attributes of the "good physician." John A. Meskauskas, M.S., another recent addition to the staff, has brought with him the benefit of his psychometric training and experience as a former member of the staff of Science Research Associates.

John R. Senior, M.D., Associate Professor of Medicine at the University of Pennsylvania, became so challenged with the potential of a computerized system for the evaluation of the clinical competence of a physician that he decided to spend a sabbatical year working toward this objective as a member of the staff of the National Board (see Chapter 12). A generous three-year research grant from the Carnegie Corporation and The Commonwealth Fund has been awarded jointly to the National Board and the American Board of Internal Medicine for support of this program.

This then is the professional staff of the National Board as of 1971. It is a unique team dedicated to the goal of measuring medical knowledge and medical competence ever more precisely. To each, I am further grateful for the careful review of this manuscript and for the comments and resulting changes that have been woven into the text.

Since the test questions are the basic substance upon which this book depends, and since every one of these questions has been prepared by the examiners of the National Board, representing both individual effort and committee review (see Chapter 2), the invaluable contribution made by these examiners must be here acknowledged. They are the authors of all questions in the large collection now in the files of the National Board; hence they are the authors of the examination questions included in this volume to demonstrate method and medical content. Their expert comprehension of the subject matter, and their prominence both in their special fields and in the broader area of medical education, are of paramount importance in maintaining the high quality of National Board examinations.

I wish to thank Dr. Barbara F. Esser for her thoughtful review of early drafts and for her helpful suggestions, Mr. Thomas R. Belvedere for his expert assistance in the design and typography of this book and Mrs. Rosemary Pattison for her skillful and understanding editing of the manuscript. Finally, I wish to express my appreciation to my secretary, Miss Brigitta Wermuth, for her diligence and perseverance as one draft followed another in the preparation of this volume.

Philadelphia   JOHN P. HUBBARD

Contents

CHAPTER 1 ▪ *The Role of the National Board of Medical Examiners*

Qualification for a Medical License

The National Board of Medical Examiners was founded in 1915 with one clear objective: to provide examinations of high quality so that the legally established licensing authorities of the states could, at their discretion, license a physician to practice without further examination.[72]* This qualification having once been established, the physician would not be confronted by state board examinations should he move from one state to another during the course of his professional career.

Until 1950 the examinations were set up as essay tests in the traditional basic medical sciences (Part I), and in the clinical-science subjects (Part II). A third part, Part III, was an oral "practical" examination. Part I was usually taken by students at the end of the second year of medical school and Part II toward the end of the fourth year. A year of internship was required for admission to Part III. Thus, as the student proceeded through his years of formal education and acquired an M.D. degree, he had the

* All references are listed in the Bibliography, pages 105 to 107. The superscript numeral in the text indicates the number of the reference in the Bibliography.

opportunity to qualify for a state license by taking and passing the three-part series of extramural examinations.

For the individual taking the examination, the point of critical importance was a passing mark. Although the examinee showed the natural tendency of students to strive for grades higher than the bare minimum for passing, the state licensing boards were really interested only in a record showing that the candidate had "passed the National Boards."* If he had passed, he could be given a license by "endorsement" of his National Board certificate without further examination; if he had failed, or if he had not taken National Boards, he must then take the examination of a state board of medical examiners.　As an increasing number of states throughout the United States recognized the high standards of the National Board, its examinations became widely accepted as a minimum standard—to be sure a respectably high but nonetheless minimum standard—for the general practice of medicine.

Thus, there came into being a system unique to the United States: the admission of physicians to the practice of their profession at the conclusion of a formal education that has built into it a series of extramural examinations the results of which are regarded by official licensing authorities as an impartial, dependable and acceptable qualification for a license to practice.[30]

Evaluation of the Process of Undergraduate Medical Education

In the early 1950s, a change was introduced with effects more far-reaching than were appreciated at the time. Objective multiple-choice testing methods had come of age. It appeared timely to marry the science of medicine to the emerging science of educational measurement. A study was undertaken with the cooperation of the Educational Testing Service to determine the applicability of multiple-choice testing methods to the field of medicine. After three years of deliberate, carefully designed experimentation, convincing evidence supported the conclusion that multiple-choice methods were superior to the time-honored essay methods for the purposes of the Board.[9,10]

Part I and Part II were converted to multiple-choice form. (Part III continued as an oral, bedside examination for another ten years until new techniques were developed for objective evaluation of clinical competence.) Each Part was reduced from three days to two days, since two days of

---

* We recognize that there are many "national boards" of examiners. Throughout this volume we will, however, refer to the National Board of Medical Examiners as the Board or as the National Board and to its examinations as the National Boards. In doing so, we are merely following popular usage throughout the medical community. We would also note that the Board is not, as its name suggests, an official governmental agency; it is incorporated as an independent organization. Further, it is not to be confused with the many boards of medical specialties.

multiple-choice tests were found to provide a much more comprehensive examination than had the earlier three days of essay tests.

Part I included a total of about 800 to 1000 multiple-choice questions in the basic medical sciences equally divided among anatomy, biochemistry, microbiology, pathology, pharmacology and physiology. Additional questions have recently been added in the behavioral sciences, recognizing the increasing acceptance of behavioral science as a basic science in the medical-school curriculum. The time allowance was 12 hours during two successive days. Thus the students were required to respond to the questions at a rate averaging approximately 75 an hour. This rate would be expected to vary considerably during the examination depending upon the length and the problem-solving nature of the questions, but at this rate most medical students found the scheduled time sufficient without an undue sense of haste or pressure.

Part II was also scheduled for 12 hours with 800 to 1000 multiple-choice questions in the clinical sciences divided equally among internal medicine, obstetrics and gynecology, pediatrics, preventive medicine and public health, psychiatry and surgery.

The change to the multiple-choice form led to precise grades free of the subjective judgments of essay examiners. In essay-test days a single examiner wrote the questions and read the thousands of essay responses. He alone determined the grade for each examination on the basis of his independent judgment of the responses. In multiple-choice testing, the correct response for each question is determined as the question is created. The scoring becomes an objective count of the examinee's responses marked on an answer sheet (see Chapter 6). Furthermore, the responsibilities for the design of the examination, the formulation of the questions and for the correctness of each question are placed upon committees of examiners; these examiners write the questions which are then reviewed, accepted, modified or rejected in outspoken, frank and free-swinging discussions in meetings of peers. For the Board's complete three-part series of examinations the number of examiners, serving on about 15 separate committees, is approximately 100. Their expert comprehension of the subject matter and their prominence both in their special fields and in the broader area of medical education are elements of prime importance in establishing and maintaining the high quality of National Board examinations.

The members of the test committees have a challenging experience as they meet together with the medical and psychometric members of the National Board staff. Furthermore, they bring back to their medical schools a deeper awareness of ways in which to evaluate the effectiveness of the educational process.

As increasing numbers of faculty members learned more about these examinations, medical schools themselves began to show a growing interest in the scores obtained by their students. The Board then began to receive requests to make its examinations available for whole classes irrespective of the individual student's interest in taking them as a qualification for a state license. Thus two categories of medical students emerged: those who elected to take the examinations as candidates for certification and those who were taking the examinations only as a requirement of the faculty. A new dimension has been created for evaluation of the educational process. Precise, reliable and useful data provided an additional measure of the effectiveness of the educational program of individual schools. Class scores for the basic-science subjects or the clinical-science subjects could be compared intramurally. Similar comparisons could be made with classes of students in other schools on a department-by-department basis, or for the basic-science subjects or the clinical-science subjects as a whole (see Chapter 7).

A subtle yet profound change in the role of the National Board began to appear gradually. No longer was the objective limited to a threshold examination for admission to the practice of medicine. The distribution of scores within a class, and the class averages, became matters of significance to the faculty as well as to the students. The scores could be used—and in many schools were used—to influence the standing of the student in his class. Mean scores of the class were studied by the faculty in relation to the curriculum in general and in detail. The examinations, having originated as an evaluation of the *product* of medical education, had become an instrument for the evaluation of the *process* of medical education.

The first comparative evaluation of medical schools based upon reliable measurements of student performance was published in 1954.[33] A more extensive description of the purposes and methods of constructing, scoring and analyzing multiple-choice examinations in medicine, and their value for group comparisons, was published in 1961.[32]

The role of the National Board at the level of undergraduate medical education has therefore become twofold: to measure as precisely as possible the current teaching in medical schools and to provide the means by which a physician may be accepted as qualified for the practice of medicine. The Board has repeatedly emphasized its conviction that its role is to measure the results and effectiveness of the educational system, not to direct it. Undeniably, there is an overlapping relationship between the educational system and the examination system. Close as that relationship is, however, the Board is on the side of the examination system. Its position is unique as a testing agency drawing its competence from highly selected leaders of the nation's medical faculty who meet together free from the responsibilities and problems of curriculum design in their own schools and departments, and whose task is to construct the instruments whereby the effectiveness of the educational system may be assessed.

This task gains added importance in the light of the pressures arising both from the public and from the medical profession for increased numbers of physicians to meet what is often spoken of as the "crisis" in the nation's health manpower. New schools are being established; existing schools are pressing toward enrollments three or four times the number thought to be maximal only a few years ago; and curricula are being cut in length. The examiners of the National Board are aware of their challenging responsibility to provide a valid basis for stability and continuing quality at a time of widespread pressures for quantity.

Evaluation at the Graduate Level

When the National Board was founded in 1915, medical education meant medical schools and what happened within them. The Flexner Report had been published a few years before[19] and the need for standards for the process of medical education had been brought into sharp focus. Standards for the product of medical education were officially the concern of the state licensing authorities. These bodies were influenced by political pressures and frequently had very little to do with the educational process. Graduate medical education was a matter of individual initiative for those who wished to pursue an academic career or to achieve preeminence in a special field of medicine.

At about the same time, in 1917, the first American specialty board was founded in the field of ophthalmology; an individual who wished to be recognized as a specialist had to meet the requirements of the American Board of Ophthalmology. Examinations were established by the Board and, before he was admitted to the examination, the candidate had to have specified years of training as a hospital resident in a program approved by the Board. In addition, he had to show evidence of experience in the specialty which was acceptable to the Board. Other specialties soon saw merit in the action initiated by the ophthalmologists and developed certifying boards of their own. Thus the pattern (one can hardly call it a system) of the American boards of medical specialties came into being. Although responsibility for the standards for the residency programs is shared with the Council of Medical Education of the AMA, the standards for requirements of years of graduate training and for the certifying examinations developed as the sole and independent responsibility of the individual boards, of which there are (as of 1971) 28 in specialties and subspecialties approved by the AMA and the American Board of Medical Specialties.[12]*

The examination procedures of the specialty boards are as variable as the boards themselves. The predominant custom has been a combination of written and oral "practical" examinations. The written examination usually serves as a screening procedure which the candidate must pass before he is admitted to the oral examination.

The first specialty board to introduce multiple-choice testing techniques was the American Board of Internal Medicine; it changed its essay tests to multiple-choice tests in 1946. In describing this change, Cecil Watson, then

* Two conjoint boards have been approved since publication of Vol. 14 of the Directory of Medical Specialists, 1969.

Chairman of the Board, stated: "I am satisfied that these examinations are superior to the essay type. They have permitted a much broader sampling of the candidate's general knowledge of internal medicine and the basic sciences pertaining thereto; as the name implies, they have been wholly objective and the correction has been correspondingly fair and uniform, which can never be with the long essay type. It has been argued that the multiple-choice examination does not probe the candidate's ability to reason as well as the essay type. This depends largely on the character of the question, which may be devised to test nothing more than factual knowledge or experience or to provide a situation which requires considerable analysis or reasoning."[70]

The experience of this specialty board with objective, comprehensive examinations was one of the factors that led the National Board to study the appropriateness of multiple-choice testing for its purposes and then to convert its written examinations to this more objective, more precise form. In 1961, by which time multiple-choice testing was overcoming initial resistance among medical educators and specialty boards, the American Board of Pediatrics asked the National Board for assistance in the preparation and scoring of its written multiple-choice examinations. Other specialty boards followed the lead of the Board of Pediatrics, and at the present time (1971) the National Board is working with 15 of the 28 Boards in the specialties and subspecialties in the design, creation, scoring and analysis of their written examinations.

This cooperative enterprise in the written examinations of the specialty boards has many advantages. Test questions that have performed well in National Board examinations are made available for specialty-board examinations, but only when such questions have been critically studied and considered by the examiners of the specialty boards to be appropriate for their candidates. Relatively few questions written for medical students are found acceptable for candidates at the graduate level. Under no circumstance is a total test designed for medical students used for qualification at the specialty level. This would violate one of the primary principles of qualifying examinations: that examinations should be designed specifically for the educational level of the examinee.

As members of the specialty boards and their examination committees became increasingly familiar with the principles and methods of educational measurement, attention was focused upon the quality and standards of the oral "practical" examination regarded as the ultimate and final determinant for certifying an individual as a specialist. In response to requests from specialty boards, the National Board has studied the oral examinations of several of them. Not surprisingly, these studies showed the effect of the variables inherent in the oral examination and a lack of reliability comparable to that which the National Board had demonstrated for its own Part III examination (see Chapter 5). As in the case of the National Board, these studies have led to modifying the oral examination or introducing more objective measures of professional competence at the graduate level. Three specialty board have requested the assistance of the National Board in introducing into their examinations the techniques developed by the National Board as objective measures of clinical competence (see Chapter 5).

Examinations as Guides to Learning

Whenever and wherever possible, examinations should be used not only as a bench mark of intellectual achievement but also as an aid to learning for the examinee. He may have spent a great deal of time in preparing for the examination. Certainly he has spent hours of concentrated effort in responding to the challenge of the examination itself. He would like to know not only where he stands in a frequency distribution of those taking the examination but also which questions he had answered incorrectly and which of the multiple choices had been agreed upon by the examination committee as the correct response. To the degree to which he is willing to accept as fact that the examiners have introduced relevant and important questions—an assumption that is by no means general—he would like to have the opportunity to learn more about those aspects of the subject where he sees for himself that he has gone wrong. In the regular examinations of the National Board (Parts I, II, and III), this type of learning experience is not available. Certain multiple-choice questions in any examination have been used in earlier examinations. If questions were returned to the examinees along with the key of correct responses, the value of these questions would be negated for subsequent examinations.*

The National Board is, however, active in other programs in which examinations are developed and used specifically as guides to learning. At the undergraduate level, examinations consisting of abbreviated composites of Parts I and II are administered to medical school classes to obtain a profile of the acquisition of medical knowledge. These examinations, made up of questions used in previous National Board examinations, contain 360 questions in equal proportion to the approximately 2,000 questions in Parts I and II. They are miniature National Board examinations, and hence have become known as "Minitests." Instead of the four days for the full certifying examinations, these Minitests are scheduled for one day. Their usefulness in providing the faculty with longitudinal guides to learning for their student classes is described in Chapter 9.

* Whenever mention is made of re-use of multiple-choice questions in National Board examinations, it should be noted that questions from one year never appear in the following year. The used questions in any examination are drawn from the extensive collection of calibrated test material (i.e., the National Board's pool described on page 9) that is an essential resource in maintaining the high quality and reliability of the Board's series of examinations. Students are repeatedly warned that any effort to try to memorize test questions reputed to be National Board questions is futile and misleading.

At the graduate level, examinations administered during the course of residency training can provide assessments of the progress of the individual trainee. In 1963, the American Board of Neurological Surgery, disturbed by the high failure rate of candidates appearing for examination for certification, approached the National Board through the Harvey Cushing Society (now the American Association of Neurological Surgeons)[21,34,57] with a proposal to study the factors leading to the high failure rate and to develop steps to reduce this rate. An examination, developed with the help of the National Board, was used as an in-training evaluation to identify and correct weaknesses in a candidate's preparation for qualification as a neurological surgeon. Test scores were reported to the candidate himself and to the director of his own training program. Trainer and trainee could then work together to strengthen any areas of weakness that had been found. The procedure was, in a very real sense, a guide to learning rather than a qualifying examination. Other programs with similar objectives have been set up with the cooperation of the National Board by the American College of Obstetrics and Gynecology and the American Neurological Association. Further detail of the manner in which these in-training examinations serve as guides to learning for those in residency training and the relationship of these programs to the qualifying examinations of the specialty boards may be found in Chapter 9.

Another application of examination methodology to the objective of self-learning has recently been initiated and has grown rapidly under the banner of "self-assessment." Specialty societies, associations, colleges and academies have as one of their major functions the postgraduate or continuing education of their members. To meet this objective, the traditional methods have been postgraduate courses and national, regional or local assemblies for lectures and discussion of advances in medicine. A new way of providing physicians with a stimulus to keep abreast of medical knowledge was introduced by the American College of Physicians in 1967. Committees of the College met with the staff of the National Board to create a series of questions for each of nine subspecialties in internal medicine. The complete series was made available for purchase by physicians, whether or not members of the College. Each participating physician received the comprehensive set of questions, made his selection of responses, sent in his answer sheets and received a report indicating those questions he had answered correctly and those he had marked incorrectly. At the same time he received references to textbooks and journals applicable to each question. He then had at hand direct and incontrovertible evidence through his own responses to indicate those areas where he had not kept up with recent advances in medicine; he also could see where even well-established principles or facts had slipped away from him. Complete confidentiality was assured. No one but himself would know how he had done on the test questions, and he himself could chart his own course of self-learning with specific guidelines to meet his needs.

This type of self-assessment and self-learning has been well received by the medical profession, and programs are being undertaken by an increasing number of specialty societies (see Chapter 10).

The National Board's Collection of Calibrated Test Material

In twenty years of developing multiple-choice questions for its own examinations and more recently in association with the specialty boards, the National Board has accumulated a large collection of test material. Questions that have stood up well when put to the test of usage have been retained in a permanent file, with full identification of the examination in which each was first used, the category of subject matter and the statistical analysis showing both the difficulty of the item and its value in discriminating between competent and less competent examinees (see discussion of item analysis, pages 32 to 35).

As pointed out earlier, the Board's two-day Part I examination consists of 800 to 1000 multiple-choice questions; Part II contains approximately the same number. Part III, being a one-day examination, has fewer items. Each year, a new examination is prepared for each Part; about two-thirds of the questions are written de novo by the Board's examination committees and one-third are drawn from the collection of previously used and calibrated questions. Also each year, questions no longer valid because of the advances in medicine and those not having performed well in the previous examination are discarded. The resulting up-to-date collection of questions (familiarly spoken of as the National Board's pool) is the resource for other examinations where the goal is to score the examinees on a scale directly related to the standards of medical education throughout the United States as reflected by performance on National Board examinations.

At a time when traditional curricula are being abandoned and new curricula introduced, at a time when the student has greater freedom to chart his own course through an increasingly broad spectrum of educational opportunities, at a time when mounting pressures for quantity of health manpower jeopardize quality, medical schools are turning to the National Board for a stable base which, because of its continuous and close relation with medical education through its rotating corps of examiners, provides standards without the accompanying ills of standardization.

If a medical school, for purposes of its own, wants to test in subjects included in Part I or Part II, or to examine comprehensively in the basic medical or clinical sciences at times other than the regular National Board examinations, the National Board will arrange to meet such requests. If a medical school wishes to study in detail the performance of its students in any major subject (or in any of the subcategories of the clinical subjects of Part II), it may obtain from the National Board a question-by-question analysis. This analysis shows the percentage of its students who answer the item correctly in comparison with the average per cent of National

Board candidates who answer the question correctly. A confidential copy of the examination questions is provided with the analysis, so that department faculties may judge the performance of their students in direct relation to the content of the examination.

For those medical schools contemplating change in their curricula or having introduced changes—and these are most of the medical schools in the United States today—a somewhat different form of examination is drawn from the pool of used material. A one-day miniature composite of Parts I and II with the same proportionate distribution of subject matter as in the complete Parts I and II, the Minitest, may be administered to one or more classes during the year in order to track the acquisition and retention of knowledge of basic medical science on the one hand and clinical science on the other. These examinations do not contain a sufficient number of questions to yield reliable subscores in individual subjects, nor are they designed for assessment of individual students. They are, however, very useful for a cross-sectional class-by-class comparison of the fund of knowledge of one class of students with that of another class at one point in time. Further, since a new form of the Minitest is created each year, it may be administered repetitively to the same class at the end of successive years to provide a longitudinal assessment of the effectiveness of the educational process.

Beyond the medical-school level, this collection of test material, calibrated against the standards of medical education in American medical schools, is the substance from which other certifying examinations are built. The examinations of the Educational Council for Foreign Medical Graduates (the ECFMG examination), those for the Federation of State Boards of Medical Examiners (FLEX), and those for the Medical Council of Canada (all described in Chapter 8) are demonstrations of the manner in which the National Board's pool of tested test questions is serving as a national resource—and to a limited extent as an international resource—for the evaluation of medical education.

Summary of Examinations

The following table shows the number of those examined by the National Board by its own examinations and those taking other examinations that the National Board helped to prepare, score and analyze during the years 1950, 1960 and 1970.

The continually expanding role of the National Board, as illustrated by the figures in the table, must have been in the mind of Nathan Womack when, as President of the National Board in 1962, he stated: "We must never forget that to the degree that we are able to measure medical knowledge, to just that same degree will medical competence be available to our people."

	1950	1960	1970
Part I: Candidates	3,598	4,775	7,221
Non-candidates	——	992	1,878
Part II: Candidates	1,810	3,357	6,410
Non-candidates	——	1,912	1,172
Part III: Candidates	1,729	2,545	5,205
Medical Schools (departmental)	——	2,312	13,509
Minitest	——	——	4,942
Specialty Boards	——	——	11,420
Licensing Authorities U.S.A. and Canada	——	1,358	4,450
FLEX	——	——	4,358
ECFMG	——	14,769	29,890
Self-assessment	——	——	2,451
In-training	——	——	1,995
Other	——	——	638
	7,137	32,020	95,539

CHAPTER 2 ■ *Test Committees and Their Tasks in Creating Objective Examinations*

The Committee Method

One of the most outstanding features of the National Board's method of creating multiple-choice examinations is test construction by carefully selected committees. These committees are made up of subject-matter specialists who meet together with the test specialists of the staff. Creative writing—and the preparation of good multiple-choice questions is one of the most exacting forms of creative writing—is not usually done best by committees. In this instance, however, experience has shown that two heads are better than one and several heads better than two.

As mentioned in the previous chapter, the Board's current corps of examiners is drawn from among the leaders of medicine and medical education in the United States and Canada. These men know medical education because they are doing it. As medical education changes they are intimately aware of the changes, because they themselves are involved in them.

Each of the major subjects of Part I and each of the major subjects of Part II are the responsibility of a separate six-man committee. Thus, six biochemists construct the test questions in their field for Part I; six pediatricians are responsible for the questions in pediatrics in Part II. Part III, on the other hand, is an interdisciplinary examination without orientation along departmental lines and is, therefore, the responsibility of interdisciplinary committees.

This corps of examiners currently includes about 100 individuals with broad geographic representation among medical schools. They serve with a rotating membership, usually for a period of four years. A committee of six has been found to be about optimal. In a smaller committee, the work falls heavily on few individuals; in a large committee, there is apt to be so much discussion that the work of the committee may suffer. With a committee of six individuals each serving four years, one member rotates off one year and two the next, replaced by carefully chosen successors; there is therefore a constant infusion of fresh talent to replace those who may have become weary of the task.

The criteria for the selection of a committee member are few but essential: (1) prominence in his field so that he can take his place at the committee table as a peer of those already on the committee; (2) commitment to medical education and its evaluation; (3) awareness of the rapid changes in the medical educational environment. It is not necessary that the newly appointed committee member have specialized experience with test techniques. His role is that of a subject-matter specialist. He will soon become familiar with the do's and dont's of test construction as the questions he submits for committee approval are subjected to the frank comments of his colleagues. Even the experienced examiner may fall into the trap of ambiguity in wording test items or he may find that, for other reasons, his test items (test questions) are not acceptable to his colleagues on the committee. He learns that every word must have precise meaning. As Lindquist has pointed out, "Few other words are read with such critical attention to implied and expressed meaning as those used in test items."[47]

Outline of Examinations

The committee begins with formulation of an outline of the intended content of the test. The purpose of this outline is to make certain that all of the important aspects of a discipline or subject are sampled and that a specified number of questions is included for each category. This procedure not only ensures a comprehensive coverage but also allows for weighting of subject matter, so that more questions can be allocated to one category and fewer to another as judged appropriate by the committee. This outline is reviewed and revised annually, to keep the test in step with changing emphases in teaching and with new concepts in medicine.

The outline is drawn up in the way that the examiners agree is best suited to their particular subject. The National Board's test committee for physiology designed an outline which, as might be expected, reflects the physiologists' viewpoint related to body functions. The outline for pediatrics was, on the other hand, approached from a very different point of view, as illustrated below:

Physiology Outline

1. Fluid and electrolyte balance, renal mechanisms
    a. Excretory functions, filtration, excretion, secretion, reabsorption, circulation, renin
    b. Body fluids, blood volume, blood-brain barrier, cerebrospinal fluid, acid-base balance, electrolytes

2. Cardiovascular physiology
    a. Cardiac electrophysiology
    b. Cardiac cycle, mechanics, and output
    c. Hemodynamics
    d. Circulation in specific organs
    e. Cardiovascular regulation
    f. Capillary exchange and lymph

3. Metabolism: energy balance, starvation, temperature regulation, fever, hypothermia, muscular exercise

4. Endocrinology and reproduction
    a. Neuroendocrine interaction: anterior and posterior pituitary controls
    b. Regulation of metabolism
    c. Reproductive biology

5. Gastrointestinal functions: digestion, hepatic mechanisms, secretions, motility, endocrine, neural control

6. Respiratory and pulmonary functions
    a. Mechanics of breathing
    b. Pulmonary gas exchange
    c. Blood gas transport and tissue gas exchange
    d. Regulation of respiration

7. General physiology: permeability, bioelectrics, secretion, contractility, mechanisms of contraction, nerve and other membrane phenomena, synaptic transmission

8. Nervous system and special senses
    a. Autonomic and somatic motor mechanisms
    b. Central integrative processes covering consciousness and other complex behavior
    c. General properties of sensory mechanisms and somatic sensation
    d. Vision, audition, and other special senses

Pediatrics Outline

1. Newborn: prenatal, premature, term
2. Growth and development: physical growth, maturation of behavior, emotional aspects, genetics and congenital anomalies
3. Infant feeding and nutritional disorders: breast feeding, artificial feeding, vitamin and mineral deficiency diseases
4. Communicable diseases: viral, bacterial, parasitic, protozoan, fungal, other; immunization
5. Systemic diseases: alimentary, respiratory, cardiovascular, genito-urinary, hematologic, neuromuscular, neoplastic
6. Metabolic disorders: endocrine, lipid, hereditary, fluid and electro-lyte
7. Therapeutics: choice of drugs, dosage, common procedures
8. Accidents: poisoning, other
9. Unclassified
10. Legal medicine

For each of the test outlines a limited number of categories of subject matter has been found to be advisable. If there are too few categories, important topics may be omitted; a large number of categories may be difficult to handle, since then there may not be enough items adequately to test each category.

Having decided upon the categories needed to cover the subject adequately, the committee determines the per cent of the total test to be allocated to each category. One category may be allocated 20 per cent of the total number of test questions, another, considered less important, may be given 5 per cent. In a test of 160 items, about the average total for one of the major subjects, a category with less than 3 per cent, or about five items, is too small to have any real meaning.

The category outline has two functions. First, it serves to remind the test committee of the areas of the subject that they have agreed upon as important. Second, the outline is distributed to all those registered for the examination so that they may have advance notice of the general content of the test; at the same time they are given examples of the form of the test questions (see Chapter 3) so that they can become thoroughly familiar with the test technique in advance and during the examination can concentrate on the content. The percentage distribution of the questions and the resulting weighting of the categories are not, however, made known to the examinees.

Comprehensive Interdisciplinary Examinations

The Part I and Part II examinations are each scheduled for two consecutive days with six hours of testing time for each day. The twelve hours for each Part are equally divided among the six major subjects, i.e., two hours each. The number of multiple-choice questions that examinees can be expected to handle during two hours varies considerably, depending upon the length of individual questions and the time required for thoughtful attention to problems presented in varying degrees of complexity (see Chapter 3). The average for the National Board's Parts I and II is usually about 75 to 80 questions per hour. Thus, each of the separate committees is responsible for introducing into the test approximately 150 to 170 multiple-choice questions. If a particular test is designed to contain a considerable number of time-consuming questions, these may be put together into a separate section of the examination with fewer questions per hour. After all, the purpose is to test the knowledge of the examinee and his ability to apply his knowledge to the problem in hand, not to see how many questions he can answer in a given period of time.

That the examination system may keep closely in step with the changing nature of the educational system, Parts I and II are set up and scored as total interdisciplinary examinations; there is no identification of individual test questions according to subject-matter areas. The grade for each Part is based on the total number of questions answered correctly rather than on an average of the grades for the component subjects. Irrespective of his performance in individual subjects, the examinee passes the Part if he answers correctly a sufficient number of questions to yield a passing score on the test as a whole (see Chapter 6). Individual subject grades have continued, however, to be reported for each of the traditional subjects for Part I and Part II, to meet the requirements of individual state licensing boards calling for specified grades in individual subjects. Also, despite protestations to the contrary, medical schools and medical students continue to manifest interest in grades in the separate subjects.

As another move to adjust to the changing and variable patterns of the curriculum, eligibility requirements for Part I and Part II were recently made more flexible; any student regularly enrolled in any approved medical school in the United States or Canada may register for either Part I or Part II at any regularly scheduled administration. The student need not wait until completion of the second year to take Part I or until his fourth year to take Part II, as had earlier been required. Thus, emphasis is placed upon acquisition of knowledge and competence rather than upon completion of predetermined periods of time.

When these changes were introduced, reactions to them were many and varied. In general, both faculty and students accepted the new comprehensive form and the scoring procedures as timely, appropriate and desirable adjustments to the variability in curriculum prevalent throughout the United States.

Students found that the interdisciplinary nature of the total examination and of individual questions was far more closely suited to their experience during the early years of medical school than would have been the previous pattern of separate tests in traditional disciplines. The newer grading procedure was in keeping with the freer use of elective time and the less formal requirement of scheduled course work. Since passing the examination became dependent only on the percentage of questions answered correctly in the total examination, students could and did compensate for weakness in certain areas with better-than-average knowledge of other areas in which they had special interest and perhaps elective work.

The Construction of the Test

The preparation of each National Board examination takes approximately one year. Each committee member writes a number of questions in accordance with the outline and with the assignment given him by the committee itself. This assignment may require an individual qualified in a particular subspecialty to write all of the questions in his area of special competence; alternatively, it may be considered preferable for the required number of questions in each category to be divided among the committee members.

One of the firmly held principles of the committee method of constructing National Board examinations is that each member of the committee will be responsible for any test item he has submitted. It is not necessary that he write the questions himself; he may enlist the help of colleagues in his department or consultants from other departments. He must, however, approve the content and the wording of each question he submits since, irrespective of the authorship, the question will be regarded as his contribution for review by the committee and he will be called upon to defend it.

(The National Board does not favor the custom, sometimes encountered in other boards or examination committees, whereby multiple-choice questions are solicited from members of the board who do not meet with an examination committee and have no further responsibility for the examination. The justification for this "mail-order" method of obtaining test questions is a desire to involve the board members or others in the specialty in the preparation of the examination. This may be good for the board member but it is not good for test construction. Too many items are received in unacceptable form and with unacceptable content, and the author of a question that may have been aimed at an important target is not there to explain what he had in mind.)

To make the submitted questions fairly uniform in style, a special form is provided to each committee member. After new items are received on this form, they are duplicated and assembled in a draft that includes not only the newly written questions but also a number of previously used test questions selected from the National Board's pool described in the previous chapter. Each of the examinations of Parts I, II, and III, therefore, contains a quota of questions tested by previous use. Both new and previously used questions are distributed to all members of the committee who are asked to study each item carefully and to determine whether it appears satisfactory as written, whether changes are indicated or whether the question is inappropriate and should be discarded. This study and criticism of individual questions are done as homework before the committee meets for a two-day session of frank, critical, around-the-table discussion of each individual item.

At these two-day committee meetings, each member of the committee is asked for comments about each question based upon his review prior to the meeting. If the question is approved by committee consensus, with or without modification, it is then marked for final draft of the test. If it duplicates another question or needs revision, it is set aside for future use. If it is judged as too difficult, too easy, inappropriate, ambiguous or for other reasons unacceptable, it is discarded altogether. Those who participate in this exercise are impressed with the value of group dynamics in arriving at final decision for acceptance or rejection of an individual test question. A far more penetrating critique arises here than through independent and individual judgment.

At this stage of their review by the committee, the questions are arranged according to categories of subject matter so that the committee members may see the content of the examination category by category. Later, when selection of the questions for final copy has been completed, the questions are rearranged by item type so that, in taking the test, the examinee encounters items of one type at one time. Then, following an appropriate set of instructions, he passes along to the next type of question, and the next, in an orderly manner. At this point, care is taken to assure that the correct responses are distributed randomly. For example, there should not be a long series in which D is the correct response, followed by another series in which B is the correct response.

As the questions are approved, discarded or set aside, consideration is given to the categories of subject matter and to the types of items. The number of items in each category is made to conform to the subject-matter outline. Attention is also given to the number of items of any one type; five is the number usually considered the minimum to justify a separate type of item under separate instructions. The selected questions are then typed and duplicated as an initial test draft. Again, inconsistencies or other faults in individual questions or in the test as a whole are noted and eliminated. Thus there are three separate occasions when each single test item is subjected to the critical review of the test committee: (1) in the homework prior to the meeting; (2) in the committee's review of the new material to be introduced into the test; and (3) in the final test draft.

Admittedly, the creation of multiple-choice examinations by committees of experts is time consuming and laborious, but free and frank discussion among colleagues produces results that cannot be achieved by any other method. Despite the exceptional qualifications of the examiners, the experience of the National Board reveals that, on the average, about one-third of the questions as originally written need revision. About one-third are discarded as too difficult, unimportant, controversial, or for other reasons not appropriate for the examination. Only about one-third of the questions originally submitted are accepted with little or no change. Consequently, confidence can be placed in the fact that each question has been thoroughly worked over and agreed upon as appropriate in content and difficulty, free from ambiguity, accurately and concisely written, and representative of important aspects of the subject.

CHAPTER 3 ■ *Types of Multiple-Choice Questions*

Three Basic Types of Questions

Twenty years ago, when the National Board of Medical Examiners converted its written examinations from essay to multiple-choice questions in cooperation with the Educational Testing Service (ETS), various types of multiple-choice questions used successfully by the ETS were adopted by the National Board. It became apparent, however, that test construction for the National Board was quite different from test construction for the ETS. The National Board, dealing with examination content specifically in the field of medicine, was relying upon panels of examiners drawn from medical school faculties who wrote the test questions themselves at home and then worked together with the Board's test experts at the conference table; most of these examiners had had little or no previous experience in creating multiple-choice questions. Certain complicated types of questions, although they had worked well in the hands of the ETS, were viewed by the National Board examiners as contrived and more likely to assess an examinee's test-taking ability than his knowledge of medicine.

After several years of experience with this relationship between the examiners who wrote the questions and the test experts at the National Board, and as a result of careful studies of the comparative values of different types of questions, the National Board cut back in the variety of types of questions that had been used in earlier days in multiple-choice examinations in medicine, as described by Hubbard and Clemans.[32] The Board now uses three basic types of multiple-choice questions. Each type has several variations and, as described in Chapter 5, new testing techniques have been introduced to provide objective measurements of clinical competence.

One-Best Response Type (Item Type A). This is the traditional and most frequently used type of multiple-choice item. (In the language of multiple-choice testing, it is customary to speak of test items rather than test questions since they are frequently presented in the form of statements rather than questions.) This type of item consists of a stem (e.g., a statement, question, case history, situation, chart, graph, or picture) followed by a series of four or five suggested answers for a question or completions for a statement. The suggested answers (completions) other than the one correct choice are called distracters.

A series of five choices (one correct answer plus four distracters) is preferred to a series of four choices. In a five-choice item, an individual knowing nothing about the subject matter has a one-out-of-five (20 per cent) chance of choosing the correct response by random guessing; in a four-choice item, his chances increase to 25 per cent by random guessing.

In this type of item (item type A), the instructions to the examinee emphasize the importance of selecting the "one-best response" from among those offered. The item usually has a comparative sense: one procedure is clearly the best out of the five choices; one diagnosis is the best among those given; one value is the most accurate response to a required calculation. In the broad field of medicine, however, contrasts are seldom sharply defined as black and white, but are apt to be varying shades of gray. In answering these questions, therefore, the examinee is instructed to look for the *best* or *most appropriate* choice and to discard others that may appear plausible but are in fact less applicable.

Here is a straightforward example of the one-best response type:

Item 1.* The most effective prophylactic agent for the prevention of recurrences of rheumatic fever is

(A) acetylsalicylic acid
(B) para-aminobenzoic acid
(C) adrenocorticotropic hormone
(D)* penicillin
(E) cortisone

* All items are numbered consecutively throughout the text. Correct responses are identified by an asterisk.

In this example the stem might have been written as a question: "Which of the following is the most effective prophylactic agent for the prevention of recurrences of rheumatic fever?" There is little advantage in an incomplete statement over a question, but the incomplete statement is sometimes preferred because it can often be expressed in a simpler way with fewer words.

In the above example, D is the correct response and those designated as A, B, C, and E are incorrect responses, or the "distracters." In the preparation of multiple-choice questions, the development of effective distracters is one of the most difficult parts of the examiner's task. Each distracter should be a plausible answer and should fit into the context of the problem at hand. Silly or implausible wrong answers should be strictly avoided. Any distracter that is obviously wrong weakens the test. If, for example, two out of five choices are so patently wrong as to present no problem to any of the examinees, the correct response becomes a one-out-of-three choice with a 33 per cent chance of a correct response by random guessing among the remaining options.

One of the criticisms often made of the multiple-choice type of test arises from having the correct response included in the question, so that the examinee may be reminded of something he might not have thought of without seeing it spelled out for him. It is not, however, necessary to name the correct response among the given choices. The above item could be written as follows:

Item 2.   The most effective prophylactic agent for the prevention of recurrence of rheumatic fever is
   (A)   acetylsalicylic acid
   (B)   para-aminobenzoic acid
   (C)   adrenocorticotropic hormone
   (D)   cortisone
   (E)* none of the above

In this manner the examinee must search his mind for the prophylactic agent most effective in the prevention of recurrence of rheumatic fever without having this agent, penicillin, suggested to him by finding it as one of the possible choices.

Again, using the above item as an example, it might be written as follows:

Item 3.   The most effective prophylactic agent for the prevention of recurrences of rheumatic fever is
   (A)   acetylsalicylic acid
   (B)   para-aminobenzoic acid
   (C)* penicillin
   (D)   cortisone
   (E)   none of the above

In this version, the "none of the above" response is incorrect and the correct response becomes C. It should be made clear to the examinee that the "none of the above" choice may sometimes be correct and sometimes incorrect. Also, when "none of the above" is used as the fifth choice, meticulous care must be taken to be sure that each choice is unequivocally correct or incorrect.

Another variant of the completion type of item is the negative form: All but one of the choices are applicable and the examinee is asked to select the one which does *not* apply, or applies *least*, or is an *exception* in some way. The following is an item of this type:

Item 4. Active immunization is available against all of the following diseases EXCEPT

    (A)   tuberculosis
    (B)   smallpox
    (C)   poliomyelitis
    (D)* malaria
    (E)   yellow fever

For a correct response to this item, the examinee must know that agents are available for active immunization against all of the diseases mentioned except malaria. This "all of the following EXCEPT," however, requires a switch from positive to negative thinking; this may throw the examinee off the track to the extent that an incorrect response might indicate a failure to follow the technique of the test rather than a true lack of knowledge of the subject. To avoid this possible difficulty, negative stems are usually placed together in a separate section of the test with special instructions calling attention to their negative form; alternately, the same subject matter may be stated positively by using the multiple true-false type of item (see page 26).

"All of the above" should not be used as a fifth distracter. Among a set of four choices followed by "all of the above" as the fifth option, it is likely that an examinee would recognize at least one as clearly incorrect. He can, therefore, eliminate not only this but the "all of the above" response and is left with a one-out-of-three choice rather than the intended one-out-of-five. Furthermore, if he knows that any two of "the above" are correct then "all of the above" *must* be the correct answer since any two correct responses among "the above" leave him no other choice for *one best* response.

The best one-out-of-five type of test item may follow, either singly or in sets, the presentation of a case history or other situation presenting a problem that can be as complex as seems appropriate to the examiner. In presenting case histories or other problem situations, a clear and concise style is urged. The objective is to give the examinee all the necessary information—but *only* the information truly necessary to make the correct response out of the choices offered. Fulsome descriptions with literary embellishments serve only to use up the examinee's time unnecessarily.

To probe several aspects of the examinee's knowledge related to a case history or problem situation, two or more multiple-choice items may follow a single stem (e.g., case history). Care should then be taken to avoid interdependence of the items, so that an incorrect response to one item does not lead to incorrect responses in all of the others. For example, the first question following a complicated case history might require the examinee to make a diagnosis. If a second item dealing with confirming laboratory procedures or therapy then follows, the examinee is in double jeopardy if he has not made the right diagnosis in answering the first question.

The following case history describes a patient with hemophilia, but the word "hemophilia" does not appear anywhere in the question. The examinee must, however, know about hemophilia in order to respond correctly to the three mutually independent questions that follow the case history.

A 14-year-old boy is admitted to the hospital with a nosebleed which followed slight trauma and which has persisted for four hours despite nasal packing. He has had repeated nosebleeds since early childhood. He had spontaneous hematuria on one occasion, and has ankylosis of both knees and the left elbow as a consequence of hemorrhage into these joints following injury. A maternal uncle was also a bleeder, but his mother, father, and two sisters have not had abnormal bleeding.

He has a blood-soaked pack in his nose and ankylosis of both knees and his left elbow. His spleen is not palpable. There is no evident lymphadenopathy; no petechiae or telangiectases are seen. The following laboratory data are reported: hemoglobin 13 gm per 100 ml; erythrocyte count 4,500,000 per cu mm; leukocyte count 12,000 per cu mm; differential count normal; platelets 460,000 per cu mm; urine shows no protein, red blood cells, or other abnormalities in the sediment.

Item 5. Which of the following tests is most likely to show an abnormality?

  (A)   Tourniquet test
  (B)   Bleeding time
  (C)* Clotting time
  (D)   Clot reaction
  (E)   Bone-marrow examination

Item 6. An abnormality would be expected in

  (A)   one-stage prothrombin time
  (B)* thromboplastin consumption test
  (C)   plasma fibrinogen content
  (D)   platelet fragility
  (E)   none of the above

Item 7. The most efficacious of the following therapeutic procedures would be

    (A) local applications of thrombin-soaked packs to the nose
    (B) intravenous administration of a suspension of fresh, normal platelets in saline
    (C)* intravenous administration of fresh plasma
    (D) intravenous administration of vitamin K
    (E) intravenous administration of fibrinogen and calcium gluconate

Other examples of the one-best choice form of item, illustrating the various ways in which this type can be used for both relatively short statements or questions and more complicated case histories and problem situations, are shown in Appendix A.

The Matching Type (Item Types B and C).* Items of a somewhat different nature may be used effectively to test knowledge of entities that may or may not be closely related. These items are particularly useful when dealing with the actions and uses of closely related drugs or the distinguishing signs or symptoms of similar diseases. A list of lettered headings is followed by a list of numbered words or phrases. For each numbered word or phrase, the examinee is required to select the one heading most closely related to it. Each heading can be used once, more than once, or not at all in the set.

In item type B, the leading list of headings may have varying numbers of entries; lists of five are preferred. Any number of items may be attached to the leading list. Care should be taken not to include items that are extremely easy or that deal with trivia merely in an attempt to get extra mileage out of the headings.

Questions 8 to 11 are examples of matching type B:

    (A) Hypertrophy of the left ventricle
    (B) Cor pulmonale
    (C) Mitral and aortic stenosis
    (D) Subpulmonic stenosis
    (E) Congestive failure without cardiac enlargement

Item   8. Long-standing silicosis (B)

Item   9. Constrictive pericarditis (E)

Item 10. Rheumatic heart disease (C)

Item 11. Systemic hypertension (A)

The leading list may have "none of the above" as an entry. Thus the candidate is challenged to think of possible associations other than those stated

*Correct responses are indicated by the letter in parentheses.

in the list. However, even more than with the use of "none of the above" in item type A, care must be taken to be sure that the association keyed as the correct response is unquestionably correct and that the numbered item could not be rightly associated with any other choice.

In another form of matching item, designated as type C, the examinee is directed to select the A response if the word or phrase is associated with A only, B if the word or phrase is associated with B only, C if the word or phrase is associated with both A and B, or D if the word or phrase is associated with neither A nor B. The following is an example:

(A) *Plasmodium vivax* malaria
(B) *Plasmodium falciparum* malaria
(C) Both
(D) Neither

Item 12. A combination of primaquine and chloroquine is the treatment of choice for an acute attack (A)

Item 13. Clinical attacks are suppressed by ingestion of chloroquine once a week while in an endemic area (C)

Item 14. Infection is prevented by ingestion of chloroquine once a week (D)

In the use of matching items, there is a temptation to add too many responses to a single stem. In the above example, three score points are involved in differentiating the features of *Plasmodium vivax* malaria and *Plasmodium falciparum* malaria. Many more items could have been included relatively easily. Therefore the examiner, especially when required to write a large number of items, should keep in mind the relative importance of the subject matter and the number of score points which a set of items of this type will contribute to the total test.

Multiple True-False (Item Types K and X). Multiple true-false items consist of a stem followed by four or five true or false statements. The stem may be in the form of a question, a statement, a case history, or clinical data presented in pictorial fashion as indicated in the sample test in Appendix A. When properly written, the multiple true-false question tests in depth the candidate's knowledge or understanding of several aspects of a disease, a process or procedure. Each of the statements or completions offered as possibilities must be unequivocally true or false, in contrast to the A type of item in which partially correct alternatives may be used as distracters. This type of question should be written so that no two alternatives are mutually exclusive, since the candidate is expected to consider the possibility that all of the choices may be correct.

One form of multiple true-false item, designated by the National Board as item type K, is characterized by a code that permits only one mark on the answer sheet so that consistency of scoring can be maintained. In another form, item type X, the examinee is instructed to respond separately to each of four or five choices so that any combination of rights and wrongs, from all wrong to all right, may be permitted. Test experts differ in their preference for item type K and item type X. Item type K is sometimes criticized as unduly complicated for the examinee, requiring him to keep the answer code continuously in mind and thus calling for more than his knowledge of medicine. Furthermore, with item type K, the examinee is confronted with an all-or-none situation. He may know something about the question but he gets no credit at all unless he responds accurately for the complete set of choices. In item type X, on the other hand, the examinee is given credit for each correct choice within the set; he gets partial credit for partial knowledge.

One advantage of item type K is that it permits unit weight for single items. Units can then be summed throughout the examination with equal weight, irrespective of the item type. This form of the multiple true-false is therefore to be preferred to type X when subscores are to be derived from interdisciplinary comprehensive examinations such as Part I or Part II of National Board examinations. If, however, the test content represented by multiple true-false items is not to be used for purposes of obtaining subscores, item type X may be preferred by the examiner as being free from the artificiality of the answer code and permitting partial credit for partial knowledge. However, studies undertaken by the National Board to compare the effectiveness and reliability of these two item types show that there is no significant difference in the rank order of the candidates when multiple true-false questions are set up in the form of item type K or item type X.

In item type K, the examinee is directed to select the A response if 1, 2, and 3 are correct; B if 1 and 3 are correct; C if 2 and 4 are correct; D if only 4 is correct; and E if all four are correct. In the following example (1) and (3) are correct; the correct response is therefore B.

Item 15. A child suffering from an acute exacerbation of rheumatic fever usually has

(1) an elevated erythrocyte sedimentation rate
(2) a prolonged P-R interval
(3) an elevated antistreptolysin O titer
(4) subcutaneous nodules

It should be noted that not only are the instructions for item type K given in detail at the beginning of any section in which this item type occurs in the test but also that the code is shown in abbreviated form at the top of every page where items of this type appear, as follows:

Directions Summarized				
A	B	C	D	E
1,2,3 only	1,3 only	2,4 only	4 only	All are correct

The above example of item type K (item 15) would read exactly the same if it were presented as item type X. The instructions to the candidate would, however, read as follows: You are to respond YES or NO to each of the four alternatives, bearing in mind that all, some or none of the alternatives may be correct. For full credit for this item, the candidate would have to answer yes to (1) and (3) and no to (2) and (4). Partial credit would be given for responses partially correct for the set, such as yes to (1) only or to (3) only. (See sample examination at Appendix A.)

Pictorial, Tabulated and Graphic Material

A single picture, roentgenogram, graph or table may be presented and a set of questions developed to deal with it. Sets of two or more closely related pictures also may be used, followed by a series of questions requiring the candidate to utilize all of the visual material in choosing his answers.

In the simplest use of pictorial material, the names of disorders, lesions, or other entities are given in the questions and the examinee is required only to match each one with the proper illustration. More is required of the examinee, however, if each question provides a brief clinical history, summary of laboratory data, or suggested therapy. He is then required to interpret the illustrations and to recognize a relationship existing between the information given and one of the illustrations. Questions accompanying graphs and charts may require the candidate to interpret the data and make certain deductions about them.

Pictorial material should clearly illustrate the point in question; it should not deal with trivia. Each question should be designed so that the examinee must refer to the visual material to arrive at the correct answer. When sets of illustrations are used and items call for a matching process, unintentional clueing (for example, a roentgenogram of a child in a series of roentgenograms where the identification of a child would give the examinee an obvious clue) is to be avoided.

For reproduction of roentgenograms or for pictorial material in color, the original transparency, that is, the original roentgenogram or 35-mm slide, provides the best quality. Glossy prints or lantern slides of roentgenograms or color prints result in less-than-satisfactory reproduction in the test booklet.

A good example of tabulated material to challenge candidates in depth in the understanding of clinical situations is shown below:

	Plasma Level mg/100 ml	Renal Clearance ml/minute	PAH Clearance ml/minute
Drug A	5	135	620
	10	130	600
	20	133	610
Drug B	5	65	612
	10	70	618
	20	68	606
Drug C	5	600	596
	10	450	604
	20	350	601
Drug D	5	600	604
	10	450	432
	20	350	354
Drug E	5	25	593
	10	60	603
	20	120	598

The above table lists the rates of renal clearance of a number of drugs in relation to their concentrations in the plasma of a human subject. All values are corrected for binding to plasma protein. The last column represents the simultaneous clearance of p-aminohippurate (PAH) at a plasma concentration permitting extraction of virtually all of the PAH in one circulation through the kidney. To answer Questions 16 to 20, select for each question the letter designating the drug which best fits the conditions described.

Item 16. Filtered by the glomerulus; partially reabsorbed by the renal tubules by a passive process (B)

Item 17. Secreted by the renal tubules by a rate-limited active transport process (C)

Item 18. Filtered at the glomerulus without tubular reabsorption or secretion (A)

Item 19. Reabsorbed by the renal tubules by a rate-limited active transport system (E)

Item 20. Secreted by the tubules but limits its own excretion by decreasing renal blood flow (D)

Good use of questions based on a graph is illustrated in Questions 21 and 22.

The graph below shows incorporation of radioactive iron in erythrocytes of peripheral blood after an intravenous injection of radioactive iron citrate. Study this graph to answer Questions 21 and 22.

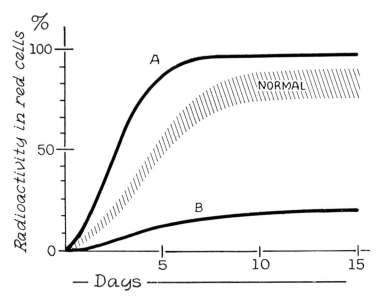

Item 21. A 40-year-old man has had prolonged gastrointestinal bleeding. He has an iron uptake as shown in curve A. This observation implies all of the following information EXCEPT

    (A)   increased erythrocyte production
    (B)   iron deficiency
    (C)* saturated iron-binding protein
    (D)   reticulocytosis
    (E)   adequate serum folic acid concentration

Item 22. A 40-year-old man has normal erythroid blood values (hematocrit 45 per cent, hemoglobin 14.6 gm/100 ml, reticulocytes 1.0 per cent). His iron uptake is shown in curve B. These findings represent

    (A)   chronic glomerulonephritis
    (B)* hemochromatosis
    (C)   agnogenic myeloid metaplasia
    (D)   congestive splenomegaly
    (E)   low serum transferrin concentration

The sample examination at Appendix A includes examples of all types of questions currently used in National Board examinations and demonstrates the use of color plates, photographs, roentgenograms and electrocardiograms.

Check List in Question Preparation

To aid the examiner in maintaining acceptable standards in the preparation of multiple-choice questions, the following check list is offered. If an item does not satisfy each of these standards, it should be discarded or revised.

1. *Does the item deal with one or more important aspects of the subject?* Minutiae of medical knowledge are to be avoided.

2. *Does the item call for information that the examinee should know or be able to deduce without consulting a reference source?* Drug dosages, limits of normal values, and other numerical data are to be included only if they deal with important information that should be within the daily working knowledge of the examinee.

3. *Is the item appropriate for the level of knowledge expected of the examinee?* Items that are too difficult or too easy cannot make effective discriminations among the examinees.

4. *Is the central problem stated clearly and accurately?* Wording that is ambiguous or fuzzy may mislead the examinee and destroy the validity of an item. All qualifications needed to provide a reasonable basis for an answer should be included.

5. *Have irrelevant clues to the correct response been avoided?* The most common clues are: the correct answer longer and more precise than the distracters, the use of common elements in stem and correct answer, inadvertent clues in grammatical construction, the use of "specific determiners" such as all, none, always, and never.

6. *Is the item written with as few words as possible to make it clear and complete?* Unnecessary words increase reading time; the examination is intended to test medical knowledge, not reading speed.

7. *Is the item type the best one for the particular point or problem?* A topic difficult to test by one type of item may be probed without difficulty by another type.

8. *Is the item written in conformity with the format?* For example, in item type A, the choices (distracters) must be grammatically consistent with the main statement (the stem) and with each other.

CHAPTER 4 ■ *Three Criteria for Multiple-Choice Questions: Difficulty, Discrimination and Relevance*

No research scientist would rely on a measurement without having been convinced about the accuracy of the measuring instrument. The same principle applies to educational measurement. A detailed analysis for each item in a test is basic to an understanding of the performance of the examinees. This chapter will, therefore, deal with the difficulty of an individual test item (the P value), the extent to which the item succeeds in discriminating between the more knowledgeable and the less knowledgeable examinees (r_{bis}), and the quality of the item in terms of its relevance to educational objectives.

Item Difficulty (P Value)

The difficulty of the individual items determines the difficulty of the test as a whole. In multiple-choice testing, the difficulty of one item is readily and precisely measurable. It is the percentage of examinees who answer the item correctly, the correct answer having been predetermined by the test committee. (The method of obtaining the index of difficulty is described below in discussion of the index of discrimination.) The higher the percentage, the easier the item. A P value of .95 would indicate that 95 per cent of the examinees responded to the item correctly and that this particular item presented very little difficulty to the examinees; nearly all knew the right answer. An item with such a high P value contributes virtually nothing to the test. It does no harm; neither does it do any good. It has the effect of giving an extra point to the examinees, good and poor alike. If, on the other hand, the P value is very low, either the item may be too difficult for the group being tested or the item itself may be defective. A choice considered wrong by the committee of examiners (a distracter) may, for one reason or another, be considered correct by a large proportion of the examinees. A P value approaching .20 for a five-choice item or .25 for a four-choice item suggests that the examinees may be indulging in chance guessing without real knowledge of the particular point or question. In such cases, the test item is carefully considered together with its index of discrimination (r_{bis}, described below) and a decision made as to whether it should be deleted from the examination in the final scoring procedure (see pages 52, 53).

In the experience of the National Board, there is a wide range of difficulty in the test items first introduced into an examination, although the average P value is usually between .60 and .65. When the examiners review the performance of candidates on individual items, they find many surprises. How could 40 per cent of medical students or residents not have known the answer to a question that the examiners had thought all should know? Sometimes an examiner goes so far as to say: "If a student does not know the answer to that question he should not pass the test!" Such an item is tagged, and the P value is brought to the attention of the examiners the following year. The examiner may then learn the fallibility of judging students on the basis of his own feelings for a single question.

The Index of Discrimination (r_{bis})

One of the objectives of any examination is to discriminate between the more knowledgeable and the less knowledgeable, between the well qualified and the less well qualified, between the good and the weak examinees— however one wishes to phrase the comparison. In evaluating National Board test items, the criterion that is used for this purpose is performance on the entire section of the test in which the particular item in question appeared. The index of discrimination employed is the biserial correlation coefficient (r_{bis}) between the item and the total score for the corresponding section of the test.*

*The biserial correlation coefficient is applicable only for large groups with a normal or near-normal frequency distribution, as in the examinations of the National Board of Medical Examiners. For determination of the discrimination index for smaller groups of examinees or groups not having a normal distribution other methods are available.[13,47]

The simplest way to calculate this discrimination index is to select a random sample of candidates, obtain a frequency distribution of their scores, identify those individuals whose scores fall in the upper 27 per cent of this distribution ("good students") and in the lower 27 per cent ("poor students"). Why use the upper and lower 27 per cent to define criterion groups? Why not select the upper and lower 10 per cent or 50 per cent? The answer is that 27 per cent provides the best compromise between two desirable but inconsistent aims: to make the criterion groups as large as possible and to make the criterion groups as different from each other as possible.[13]

The size of the sample chosen for this analysis is typically 370 examinees. A larger sample size would have little practical value in terms of improving the precision of the statistics. With a sample of this size and 27 per cent of this sample selected for a criterion group, the criterion group has 100 examinees (27 per cent of 370 is 100). Thus the subsequent arithmetic is facilitated and it is an easy matter to determine the percentage of students answering each item correctly in each criterion group. With these percentages in hand, the r_{bis} and the P value for each item can be obtained directly from published tables.[16]

The index of discrimination provides a useful measure of the difference in the knowledge of the examinees that an individual test item can contribute to the examination. If all of the top 27 per cent respond correctly and if none of the bottom 27 per cent respond correctly, the r_{bis} would be 1.00. This would then be a perfect item in terms of its ability to discriminate, but this ideal is never achieved in examinations such as those of the National Board. If equal numbers of the two groups respond correctly, the r_{bis} index is zero, indicating complete lack of discrimination. If the item is responded to correctly by more of the bottom group than of the top group, the r_{bis} index is negative and something is wrong with the item. Usually the defect is to be found in the fact that one or more of the distracters appeared more attractive to the examinees than the choice agreed upon by the examiners as the correct answer.

Since the discrimination index is a measure of difference between the top and bottom groups, it follows that the more nearly alike—the more homogeneous—these groups are, the lower the r_{bis} of a test item. Conversely, when an item with a relatively low discrimination index in an examination for U.S. medical students is used in an examination for a more heterogeneous group, as for example graduates of foreign medical schools, the r_{bis} index may be much higher. The top group and the bottom group are more different and a sharper discrimination is more readily achieved.

Item analysis data for each of the items used in National Board examinations are maintained in its pool of items. The following is a typical example pertaining to Question 4 in the clinical examination, q.v. page 133:

Item 4. A patient with a history of fever and mild diarrhea of two months' duration is found to have a palpable mass in the right lower quadrant of the abdomen. The most likely diagnosis is

(A)* regional enteritis
(B) ulcerative colitis
(C) amebic colitis
(D) diverticulitis
(E) lymphoma

	*A	B	C	D	E	P	r
High	80	2	6	6	6		
						.59	.45
Low	36	4	9	17	34		

In the above example the five possible choices for the item are indicated by the letters A to E. In the item analysis appearing below are two rows of numbers under the letters designating the responses. The top row of numbers shows the percentages of examinees in the high group who responded to the indicated choices; the lower row gives the same information for the low group. For this item, A is the correct response, indicated by a *. The P value is .59, or the percentage of candidates answering the item correctly in the total group. The r_{bis} is .45. The item was moderately difficult for the average student. It discriminated very well between the high and low groups, with each of the distracters (wrong answers) having some responses among both the high and low groups.

In the experience of the National Board, an r_{bis} of .25 is considered acceptable. Higher values are desirable but r values higher than .50 are seldom attained in the field of medicine. An r_{bis} less than .15 indicates an item of doubtful quality. The r value is studied together with the P value, the responses to the distracters, and a critical review of the wording of the stem. As mentioned in relation to the P value, a low value in the chance range is in itself cause to consider deleting an item from the test. If, however, a low P value is coupled with a satisfactory r_{bis}, and if a critical review of the item suggests no defect in its content or wording, it may be concluded that the item should be retained as a very difficult item, having the effect of discriminating at the high end of the scale between the "good" and the "very good" examinees.

The Relevance of Test Items

The relevance of test items to the objectives of medical education is a factor that does not lend itself to expression in numerical values. It is a judgmental concept related to what the examiner thinks the examinee should know and is subject to interpretations of the aims of medical education and of the degree to which a particular question or problem may be directly related to such aims. The range of such interpretations is wide and growing wider as the educational system endeavors to adjust to the massive quantity of medical knowledge and to decide what, from this overwhelming mass, should be included in the medical school curriculum.

The resulting uncertainties and changing curricular patterns create a formidable challenge for the examination system. The National Board's answer to this challenge lies in the collective judgment of its corps of examiners—about 100 representatives of the educational system. However, even the judgment of 100 distinguished medical educators currently active in the educational process on a national basis may be questioned by an individual medical school.

Repetitive studies have been undertaken by the National Board to determine the degree to which the grades resulting from its examinations do in fact agree with the independent judgment of medical school faculties in ranking their own students. At the very outset of the National Board's use of multiple-choice tests during the academic year 1952-53, medical schools in which all or nearly all students were then taking National Board examinations were asked to provide, prior to the examinations, ratings of the proficiency of students in the subjects of the tests. These ratings were simply listings of students designating the top fifth, middle three-fifths and lower fifth of the class in each subject. As reported by Cowles and Hubbard,[10] correlations of test scores and faculty ratings were very satisfactory, demonstrating that the results of these early National Board examinations did correspond closely with the appraisal of students by their own faculties. Similar studies have been carried out subsequently with larger numbers of participating medical school classes; they are described in Chapter 6, pages 56, 57.

During the academic years 1969-70 and 1970-71, a different approach to determining the judgment of the medical educational community about the validity and relevance of National Board examinations was undertaken.* The Board committed itself to a rather bold and forthright undertaking: to ask and to answer, for all to see, how National Board examinations fit the educational objectives of medical schools. A further question could have been asked: whether the educational objectives are adequately oriented to the needs of society. Exploration of this latter question, however, was not viewed as the task of the National Board. The Board's function remains that of measuring fully and fairly what is being taught in medical school today, leaving to others the determination of what ought to be taught.

The data resulting from this study were, on the whole, reassuring: 90 per cent of the questions in the basic medical sciences were judged by two-thirds or more of the basic-science departments to represent important knowledge relevant to their disciplines. The view of clinical faculties when

* The National Board of Medical Examiners is indebted to the Carnegie Corporation and The Commonwealth Fund for financial support for this research study.

they too judged basic-science questions was expectedly variable. Nevertheless, 83 per cent of the questions in basic medical science were considered relevant by one or more of the clinical departments. A similar assessment of clinical-science questions by clinical departments also gave a reassuring view of the relevance of individual clinical-science questions.

A question closely related to that of relevance of individual items deals with what the items are really measuring. A frequent criticism of multiple-choice examinations is that they place a premium on memorization and factual recall. This pitfall was recognized when the Board first introduced multiple-choice questions into its national examination. It came into sharp focus when the first examination committee met in 1951 to formulate a multiple-choice examination in pharmacology. This committee decided that intellectual exercises such as memorizing drug doses were not in the best interests of medical education and should not, therefore, be a feature of the test unless the knowledge was considered important enough to be in the mind of the well-qualified physician without recourse to reference sources.

(This first committee was so enthusiastic about its task and found the writing of good multiple-choice questions so exciting that it worked not only through the day but through the evening and until three o'clock the next morning, thereby demonstrating for the benefit of all subsequent committees that multiple-choice questions created after midnight do not look very acceptable the next day. Thereafter, each of the Board's test committees was scheduled for a working session of two and sometimes three consecutive days.)

As the examiners of the National Board gained experience and as the examinations gained acceptance by medical schools and licensing authorities, they were not, however, without their critics. In a study reported by McGuire,[50] selected members of the faculty of the University of Illinois College of Medicine were asked to apply to each question in a National Board examination "an eight level classification of intellectual processes" adapted from Bloom's *Taxonomy of Educational Objectives*.[3] The faculty judges were instructed to "determine by introspection what intellectual process a student would be required to use in order to answer the question." Did it require only recall of factual information? Did it depend on the meaning of a fact or principle? Did it call for interpretation of data or solution of a specific problem or—and this is the highest order in the taxonomy—did it require synthesis of data? The conclusion of the author, based upon the subjective opinions of the faculty members participating in the study, was that National Board examinations "measured recall of isolated information."

This study is itself subject to criticism, for several reasons. The Bloom taxonomy is, as Bloom himself clearly states,[3] intended for use by a teacher who knows very well what each student has been taught and who can therefore classify with reasonable accuracy the cognitive process needed to answer a specific question. To attempt to determine the mental process of a student of medicine when confronted with a test question or problem on a national examination, when the examiner has no possible way of knowing what the student may have learned about the particular question or problem, is a very different matter. A situation which is complicated for one student may be a matter of simple recall for another who has learned all about it.

Robert Ebel[14] has sounded a timely warning in discussing the taxonomy of educational objectives in relation to National Board examinations. As he points out, "Terms like translation, interpretation, extrapolation, analysis, synthesis and evaluation are useful general terms for some related kinds of specific activity. But we should beware of the semantic trap of assuming from the use of a single term that a single ability is responsible for the varied activities."

John Hickam, when Professor of Medicine at the Indiana University School of Medicine, gave his view of this issue as follows:[28]

> The statement that the National Board examinations test predominantly simple recall and the implication that they may therefore be unsatisfactory deserve further consideration. First, the present data indicate that National Board grades in medicine correlate well with student performance in actual clinical situations. In the second place, it is essential that a practicing physician have a large store of modern information at his fingertips. Unless he has this he cannot define the problem which a patient presents in terms of present-day medical concepts, nor can he determine what additional information he may need to decide on a course of action. The ability to solve problems, however desirable, cannot compensate entirely for a submarginal stock of information. In the third place, the intellectual process which makes the appropriate information available is not necessarily "simple." Every medical student is exposed to much more information than he can remember. He makes an effort to retain only that information which he perceives as being important. This information is not retained by the usual student as an accumulation of isolated facts but as facts which fit into some kind of pattern and are related to one another. To the experienced clinical teacher who works often with students at the bedside it is a familiar observation that the student who can make connections and solve problems is also the one who is most successful at remembering pertinent facts. In clinical medicine the processes are not as dissimilar as they might seem. In brief, facts are of great importance to a physician, and the ability to accumulate medical information selectively, relevantly, and economically and to bring forth what is appropriate to a particular situation is different from the kind of recall involved in remembering the multiplication tables. Finally, coming up with a particular bit of information may be simple remembering for one individual because of extreme familiarity but may require complex

problem-solving for another who has available as starting points only some distantly connected facts.

The present data indicate that the present National Board medicine test stands up well as an index of the performance to be expected from students in clinical situations.

Although skeptical about the validity of the taxonomy classification of its test items, the National Board staff undertook a study of the performance of National Board candidates on those test items classified by McGuire as low taxonomy (level 1) and high taxonomy (levels 3 to 7). Basic to the taxonomy approach is the concept that different items require different intellectual processes. Identifiable differences should therefore be observable between the performance of examinees on low- and high-taxonomy items.

After combining the data for Parts I and II, of National Board examinations, the average correlation between scores on the low-taxonomy items and the total test score was .25. The average correlation between scores on the high-level items and the total test score was .28. Thus there was no significant difference between the high- and low-level items in terms of average correlation with scores on the total test. Further evidence of lack of difference between high- and low-level taxonomy items was provided by high positive correlations (.73 for Part I and .83 for Part II) between scores on low- and high-taxonomy items. Still further lack of difference resulted from a correlation between low-level items and high-level items against scores on the Part III examination, which features problem solving, synthesis of diagnostic information about a patient, and judgment in his management. The taxonomy concept would suggest that high-level items in Part II would show a higher correlation with Part III scores than would those items judged to fall in the recall category. No significant differences were found between high- and low-taxonomy items in terms of average correlation with total score on Part III; the correlations were .11 and .15 respectively.

These observations are not intended in any way to deny the importance of assiduous and constant attention to the creation of items that are in fact relevant to the sound educational objective of probing the candidate's knowledge in depth and his ability to apply that knowledge to the question or problem before him. They do, however, seem to indicate the futility of trying to categorize test items in a national examination according to a neatly compartmentalized hierarchy of cognitive processes.

CHAPTER 5

■ *Objective Evaluation of Clinical Competence*

Ever since the beginning of National Board examinations, one part of the total procedure—a final Part III—has been included for the purpose of evaluating clinical competence. Before 1961, Part III was conducted as an oral bedside examination. After completing a history and physical examination of an assigned patient, the candidate was questioned by an examiner who was perhaps unfamiliar with the patient and who would, using the patient's chart, develop the examination along the lines of a quiz session that was an inadequate test of knowledge—the candidate's knowledge already having been more thoroughly tested in Parts I and II. The procedure would then be repeated at a second bedside, with another patient and another examiner. "Clinical competence" at the two bedsides might be, and often was, evaluated quite differently from examiner to examiner. The bedside evaluations were influenced by three variables: the examiner, the patient, and the candidate. The increasingly apparent problem was how to control two variables, the examiner and the patient, in order to obtain a reliable measurement of the third variable, the one of critical interest, the candidate.

In 1959, the National Board undertook to analyze and define the clinical competence its Part III was intended to measure, and to devise testing techniques permitting objective, valid and reliable assessments of clinical competence as thus defined.[31,35] A two-year study was initiated with the co-operation of the American Institute of Research and its Director, Dr. John Flanagan, who had successfully developed objective methods for measuring skills of airplane pilots—another critical area of human responsibility.[17,18,22]*

Definition of Clincal Competence

The first step in this research project was to obtain a definition of clinical competence and skill at the level of the internship, as the young physician with his M.D. degree begins to assume independent responsibility for the care of patients. The method used was "the critical incident technique."[18] By interview and by mail questionnaires, senior physicians and residents, all of whom had direct responsibility for supervision of interns, were asked to record clinical situations (incidents) in which they had personally observed interns exhibiting, in their judgment, good clinical practice on the one hand and conspicuously poor clinical practice on the other. A total of 3300 incidents was collected from approximately 600 physicians. These incidents were divided about equally between "good" and "poor" practice. A review of these records provides an interesting—and also disturbing—description of actual behavior during internship. Among the most frequently reported examples of good clinical practice were the following: taking a history thoroughly and performing a physical examination in a systematic way; accurately recognizing the patient's condition from observation of clinical signs; withholding decision about diagnosis until all needed information was available; correctly suspecting an obscure diagnosis despite obvious symptoms and signs of another condition; and taking appropriate emergency action when indicated.

In contrast, the most frequently recorded examples of poor or inappropriate clinical practice were as follows: failing to consider other than the most obvious causes of symptoms and signs; making a diagnosis with inadequate information; and prescribing medication with inadequate indication.

The information resulting from the 3300 incidents was reduced to manageable proportions; the incidents were summarized individually, grouped and classified. They fell into nine major areas of clinical performance, with subheadings as follows:

    I. History:
        A. Obtaining information from patient.
        B. Obtaining information from other sources.
        C. Using judgment.

* The National Board gratefully acknowledges a generous research grant from the Rockefeller Foundation in support of this project.

II. Physical Examination:
   A. Performing thorough physical examination.
   B. Noting manifest signs.
   C. Using appropriate technique.

III. Tests and Procedures:
   A. Utilizing appropriate tests and procedures.
   B. Modifying test methods correctly.
   C. Modifying tests to meet the patient's needs.
   D. Interpreting test results.

IV. Diagnostic Acumen:
   A. Recognizing causes.
   B. Exploring condition thoroughly.
   C. Arriving at a reasonable differential diagnosis.

V. Treatment:
   A. Instituting the appropriate type of treatment.
   B. Deciding on the immediacy of the need for therapy.
   C. Judging the appropriate extent of treatment.

VI. Judgment and Skill in Implementing Care:
   A. Making necessary preparations.
   B. Using correct methods and procedures.
   C. Performing manual techniques properly.
   D. Adapting method to special procedure.

VII. Continuing Care:
   A. Following patient's progress.
   B. Modifying treatment appropriately.
   C. Planning effective follow-up care.

VIII. Physician-Patient Relationship:
   A. Establishing rapport with the patient.
   B. Relieving tensions.
   C. Improving patient cooperation.

IX. Responsibilities as a Physician:
   A. For the welfare of the patient.
   B. For the hospital.
   C. For the health of the community.
   D. For the medical profession.

These nine major areas with their subdivisions, derived from factual information drawn from actual performance, constituted a well-documented answer to the question of *what* to test. The next step—and a formidable one—was to determine *how* to test designated skills and behavior of interns. Many methods were explored: motion pictures, television, lantern-slide projection, various forms of the "tab test," and the technique developed by Rimoldi[60] to test diagnostic skills and reported by him in a series of papers.

At first these techniques were looked upon as possible supplements to, rather than substitutes for, the traditional bedside examination, long considered the ultimate in testing the competence of a physician. Therefore, in addition to the introduction of the new methods described below, an attempt was made to improve the reliability of the bedside examination. An evaluation form was carefully devised for an examiner to complete as he watched the candidate taking a history and performing the physical examination. This form was also intended to standardize the oral examination directly related to the patient. As the candidate proceeded to a second patient and a second examiner, another copy of the same evaluation form was used. This method was used over a three-year period as a part of the examination; analysis of the results, however, indicated that it had not resolved the problem of the two variables examiner and patient, and did not therefore yield a reliable measurement of the third variable, the candidate. A study of the correlation between the independent evaluations of a single candidate made by the two examiners showed that agreement was still only at the chance level ($r = 0.25$ for a total of 10,000 examinations). The bedside examination was therefore discontinued after 1963.

The medium of motion pictures appeared to offer an objective method of testing many of the areas of clinical competence defined by the critical incidents study. In motion picture films a patient can be shown to all examinees at the same time. Questions about observable signs and features of the patient can then be asked in multiple-choice form. If sound accompanies the motion picture, a dialogue between physician and patient can be introduced to test the examinee's knowledge about skill in taking a clinical history and communicating with the patient. Auscultatory signs can be and have been included for testing purposes. In the experience of the National Board, however, the use of motion pictures, with or without sound, has failed to yield tests meeting the Board's high standards for certification examinations. Unquestionably motion pictures have gained a firm place in the educational system for purposes of teaching, but it is doubtful that they will be continued as a feature of National Board examinations in the same form in which they have been used since 1961. It is more likely that motion pictures will be supplanted by other methods as computer technology advances and is coupled with projection capabilities for pictorial material and possibly linked to videotape or even to television (see Chapter 12).

Programmed Testing of Patient Management Problems

A new and different testing method was devised and introduced by the National Board for the first time in 1961 to test aspects of clinical competence dealing with the ability to identify, to resolve and to manage patient problems.[31,35] This method simulates a realistic clinical situation in which the physician must face the dynamic challenge of a sick or injured patient. As in real life, the candidate is confronted with a patient about whom he may have limited information. He must study the available information, and then he must decide what to do. He may require laboratory studies and diagnostic procedures; he must arrive at decisions about therapy and management. In the test booklet, a list of possible procedures immediately follows the description of the patient. Some of these procedures are correct and mandatory for the proper management of the patient; others are incorrect or contraindicated. The candidate is not told how many procedures or courses of action are considered correct; his task is to select those he judges to be indicated at this point in time. After he has decided upon a course of action, he is instructed to turn to a separate answer booklet where he finds a series of inked blocks, each block numbered to correspond to one of the given choices. He removes the ink for his selected choice with an ordinary pencil eraser, and the result of his decision appears under the erasure. He is told that information will appear under the erasure for incorrect as well as correct choices; if he has ordered a diagnostic test, the result of the test will appear under his erasure whether or not the selected test should have been ordered.

As the examinee makes his erasures he gains information from his decisions, from the courses of action he has selected. The situation changes: a new problem evolves and new decisions and actions are called for in the light of new information and altered circumstances. A second series of choices constitutes a second problem; again the candidate reaches his decision and turns to the answer booklet to discover, by erasing the appropriate ink blocks, the consequence of his second series of decisions. He continues in this manner through some four to six problems (sets of given choices of action) following the patient's course for days, weeks, or months, until the patient improves and is discharged from the hospital, or possibly dies.

This step-by-step progression, each step accompanied by an increment of information upon which the next step depends, is the characteristic feature of this testing method, which, because of its similarity to programmed teaching, led to the designation of this technique as "programmed testing." In programmed teaching the basic characteristic, with or without teaching machines, appears to be a step-by-step progression toward carefully constructed goals. Each step calls for specific knowledge. The student must have the knowledge, or he must master it, before he can progress to the next step. Similarly, in this programmed testing method, the examinee proceeds in a step-by-step fashion through a sequential unfolding of a series of problems. And, as in programmed teaching, additional information essential for the handling of the problem is concealed until the examinee has made his decision and thus earned the right to have the information.

At first there was considerable difficulty in finding a printing technique permitting erasure of the overlying ink without, at the same time, erasing the underlying information. After considerable trial and error a satisfactory method was developed by laminating a thin acetate layer on the pages containing the answer. Blocks of ink were applied over the acetate layers to cover the underlying printing. The ink is of a special formula so that, when dry, it can be removed readily by an ordinary eraser. The acetate layer protects the underlying printing.

The programmed testing method is readily adaptable to mass testing and is foolproof for scoring purposes. The examinee has no way of replacing the ink over an answer once he has erased it. If, when he sees the result of his decisions, he finds that he has made a wrong choice, or if mistaken choices become apparent as the solution to the problem gradually unfolds, he is stuck with the choices he has made. He cannot change his answers and he cannot cheat by peeking ahead as he might if the answers were covered with tabs or printed on the back of a series of cards.[60] His responses, whether right or wrong, are clearly apparent for the scorer to count.

When this technique is used in an examination, the examinee is given an opportunity to try his hand at an oversimplified example to familiarize himself with this method of testing.

Figure 1 shows the back page of a test booklet. Before breaking the seal of the booklet, the examinee is given a chance to practice on two simplified sample problems related to one patient. A brief paragraph describes a patient brought to the emergency room of the hospital in coma. From the information given, any intern would recognize the coma as due to diabetes. The first problem for this patient then offers six courses of action calling for immediate decision. Three of these six choices (2, 4, and 6) constitute proper management at this point; selection of these three and only these three choices leads to a perfect score for this problem.

Figure 2 shows the answer blocks for choices 3, 4, and 5 in this list. Choice 4 is one of the essential procedures. The erasure has been made and the answer revealed. The examinee has decided to catheterize the patient to test the urine, and the urine is found to contain large amounts of sugar and acetone, characteristic of the condition with which the candidate is dealing. If he did not recognize diabetes as the cause of the patient's coma and selected choice 5, to perform a lumbar puncture, his erasure for this choice would reveal the word "scheduled." Thus, in very realistic fashion, the situation simulates that with which an intern might be confronted when the decisions are entirely his own with no senior physician to advise him. He makes his own decision and obtains the results of his action.

Having made his decisions for the immediate steps to be undertaken for this patient, the candidate then proceeds to the second problem. Figure 3 shows the answer blocks for items 7, 8 and 9 appearing in this second problem. Item 9 reads "order insulin." This is a correct decision, arising from the information that he should have uncovered in the first problem;

SAMPLE PATIENT

A 40-year-old man with known diabetes is brought to the hospital in a comatose state. There is no obvious evidence of trauma. There is Kussmaul breathing and the breath has an acetone odor. The eyeballs are soft to palpation. Examination of the heart and lungs shows nothing abnormal except for labored respiration and a rapid, regular heart rate of 120 per minute. The abdomen is soft. There is no evidence of enlarged liver or spleen or abnormal masses. Deep tendon reflexes are somewhat hypoactive bilaterally. The rectal temperature is 36.7 C (98.0 F). Blood pressure is 100/70 mm Hg.

SAMPLE PROBLEM S-1

You would immediately

1. Order serum calcium determination
2. Order serum bicarbonate determination
3. Measure venous pressure
4. Order urinalysis (catheterized specimen)
5. Perform lumbar puncture
6. Order blood glucose determination

SAMPLE PROBLEM S-2

You would now

7. Administer digitalis
8. Administer morphine
9. Administer insulin
10. Administer coramine
11. Start intravenous infusion with normal saline

INSTRUCTIONS
FOR SAMPLE PATIENT

1. First study the initial information given.

2. Read all of the courses of action given in Problem S-1. Then select a study or procedure that you consider pertinent and necessary and erase the blue rectangle numbered to correspond to this choice. (In the actual test, these appear in the separate answer booklet.) The information you receive may lead you to select other procedures within this problem, or you may decide to make other choices quite independent of results already obtained.

3. After you have completed Problem S-1, and bearing in mind the additional information resulting from your decisions, proceed in a similar manner with Problem S-2.

4. In this simplified example of a patient with diabetic coma, the correct actions in Problem S-1 are 2, 4, and 6; in Problem S-2, the correct actions are 9 and 11.

5. In this sample, as in the actual examination, responses are given for incorrect as well as for correct courses of action.

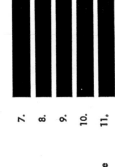

ANSWER BOOK

Fig. 1.

3. Measure venous pressure   3.

4. Order urinalysis (catheterized specimen)   4.

5. Perform lumbar puncture   5.

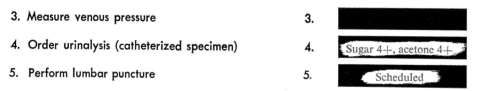

Fig. 2.

he erases the corresponding inked block and sees that insulin is ordered as a result of his decision. He is also given the opportunity to order other medication as, for example in item 7, digitalis. This is an incorrect choice reflecting error in the first problem; if he should order digitalis, he would find, as revealed under his erasure, that digitalis is given in accordance with his orders. In the actual internship situation, it might not be until the following morning, when the patient is seen by the Chief of Service, that the intern learns of his error in administering digitalis.

7. Administer digitalis   7.

8. Administer morphine   8.

9. Administer insulin   9.

Fig. 3.

This example of a patient with diabetic coma, oversimplified for purposes of demonstrating the test technique, gives no adequate representation of the test content in the actual examination. Examples of more complicated patient management problems (PMP), taken from National Board examinations, are to be found in the sample examination at Appendix A.

Scoring Patient Management Problems (PMP)

The scoring of patient management problems gives credit for correct decisions and penalties for sins of omission and commission. Each of the several hundred choices, or courses of action, offered in the test is classified in one of three categories: (1) it must be done for the well-being of the patient; (2) it should definitely not be done and, if done, would be a serious error in judgment that might be harmful to the patient; and (3) it is relatively unimportant, i.e., a procedure that might or might not be done, depending upon local conditions and customs. Each examinee is given a "handicap score" equal to the total number of items coded as definitely incorrect. Each time the examinee selects an incorrect choice, one point is subtracted from this score; each time he selects a correct choice, one point is added. Thus, his total score on this test is the number of correct decisions he has made, i.e., the number of indicated procedures he has selected plus the number of incorrect procedures that he has avoided. The choices in the equivocal middle ground receive no score.

The programmed testing method is quite different from the usual multiple-choice technique in which the candidate is offered a number of choices and instructed to select one best response. Here, he is offered a number of choices and required to use his best judgment in selecting all those, and only those, he considers important for the management of the patient. Usually, as in a practical situation on a hospital ward, he recognizes a number of actions that should definitely be done and other actions that should definitely not be done. His responses are therefore interrelated. If he is on the right track, he makes a number of correct decisions from among the available choices; then, by his erasures, he gains the information necessary for the proper management of the patient in the next problem and in the next set of choices. If he starts off on the wrong track in this programmed test, he may compound his mistakes as he proceeds and become increasingly dismayed as he learns from his erasures the error of his ways. If he discovers that he is on the wrong track, however, he has a chance to change his course and to make additional choices, although he cannot undo the errors that he has already committed—again a situation rather true to life.

Since in this testing technique, as in the use of the more traditional type of multiple-choice examinations, a panel of experts has determined the rightness or wrongness of each choice or course of action offered to the examinee, accurate and detailed statistical analyses are equally applicable. The essential criterion of test reliability will be dealt with in Chapter 6. Here it suffices to say that the reliability of the programmed testing section of Part III is generally at the level of .80 to .85,[*] which compares favorably to a section of equal length in Part I or Part II despite the fact that, in the desire to simulate real-life situations, interrelated responses are included within each problem and between one problem and the next. This interdependency has the effect of decreasing the number of points upon which the test score is built and, consequently, decreases the reliability of the test.

This programmed testing of patient management problems has also been studied to determine the extent to which it is in fact measuring something different from that which has already been measured in the comprehensive examinations in the basic medical sciences (Part I) and the clinical sciences (Part II). Unless significant differences could be found, this portion of the examination would have added nothing to the assessments of the candidates already made. Correlations were, therefore, calculated between the PMP section of Part III and Part II; the correlations ranged from .34 to .48. These correlations, positive yet moderate, reflect the degree of correlation that would be expected between medical knowledge and addi-

---

[*] The reliability of the total, full-day Part III examination, consisting of clinical material presented in graphic and pictorial form as well as the PMP section, is approximately .90.

tional elements of clinical competence inevitably based upon medical knowledge but representing skills that are to a degree independent of factual knowledge. If these correlations were high, they would have indicated that the patient management problems were measuring the attributes already thoroughly measured, and the test would be superfluous.

As illustrated by the oversimplified example of a patient in diabetic coma, and as demonstrated more fully by the patient management problems included in the sample examination in Appendix A, this programmed testing technique may be likened to the linear method of programmed teaching rather than to the branching program method. Although the branching program method may seem attractive, and has been introduced by McGuire[50] as a modification of the PMP test, the National Board has held to the linear method to assure that each examinee is tested with essentially the same examination. When unlimited branching is permitted, two different examinees may take totally different approaches to the clinical situation and follow different pathways to the solution of the problem. In this case there is no accurate way to evaluate the two examinees except in terms of whether or not they ultimately solved the problem (e.g., gave the "correct" final diagnosis) regardless of what they had done (or not done) for the patient in the interim.

Failure on Part III

Who are the failures in Part III? Why should individuals fail, having acquired an M.D. degree in an approved medical school in the United States or Canada? Why should such individuals fail after having passed the Board's comprehensive examination in the clinical subjects (Part II) and in the basic medical sciences (Part I)?

In an attempt to answer these questions, scores of 145 candidates who failed a PMP examination were studied to determine the types of errors made. As pointed out earlier, in this examination it is possible to make two kinds of errors: errors of commission (choosing courses of action harmful to the patient), and errors of omission (failing to choose the courses of action beneficial to the patient). Theoretically, the poorest possible score on this test could be obtained by committing both of these types of errors, i.e., ordering all of the contraindicated measures and failing to order anything of benefit to the patient. However, none of the 145 candidates who failed the test behaved in this manner. Rather, the failures fell at either end of another dimension, apparently related to the number of decisions made. One type of failure is the "shotgunner" who orders a large number of studies or procedures. He commits relatively few errors of omission but, at the same time, he orders so many contraindicated procedures that even the most hardy patient would have difficulty in surviving. The other type of failure is the timid soul who makes very few choices lest he make a mistake. This candidate rarely makes an error of commission; his failure is in omitting procedures beneficial for his patient, and possibly even life-saving.

These two types of young physician, the "shotgunner" and the timid soul, were quite clearly identified by the critical incident study forming the basis for the development of the PMP test. As noted in that study, the most frequently recorded examples of poor or inappropriate clinical practice observed among interns included: making a diagnosis with inadequate information (the timid soul) and prescribing medication with inadequate indication (the shotgunner). It is these physicians who, as failures on Part III, are judged by the National Board as not yet ready to be licensed for the practice of medicine, with full responsibility for the care and well-being of patients.

CHAPTER 6 ■ *Scoring and Analysis*

CHARLES F. SCHUMACHER

This chapter describes the scoring procedures and psychometric analyses applied to National Board examinations after they have been administered to large groups of examinees. No attempt has been made to describe or even enumerate all techniques of scoring and analysis; these may be found in many excellent texts on psychometric methodology.[2,13,25,26,32,47,69] The methods currently being used by the National Board will be described in the light of twenty years of experience and continuous study. The concepts of reliability, validity, score conversion and intercorrelation among test scores will be reviewed as they pertain to the series of National Board examinations, rather than as abstract psychometric principles.

This chapter will also describe the process of setting standards such as passing levels, a process that goes beyond the realm of psychometrics but uses psychometric information as a basis for decision-making.

Scoring

As pointed out earlier, the rightness and wrongness of each response to multiple-choice questions is predetermined by the panel of subject-matter specialists who write the questions and approve them for inclusion in the examination. The examinee makes his choice of the correct response as he takes the examination and records this choice on a special answer sheet. The first step in scoring is then to count the correct responses. Various scoring machines are used, depending in part upon the number of answer sheets to be scored and the urgency with which results must be reported. If very few individuals, or possibly a single individual, are to be examined, machine scoring may not be justified and the scoring may then be done by hand. Template forms are available or may be designed to provide for holes to be punched over the location of the correct response on the answer sheet. It is then an easy matter to count the correct responses appearing through the holes.

For the scoring of any multiple-choice test, a decision must be made as to which scoring formula will be used. When the examination is one in which all, or nearly all, examinees are given enough time to consider every item and are encouraged to record an answer for each item based upon whatever information they may have, the problem of selecting a scoring formula is largely academic. In this situation, scores based upon the number of questions answered correctly will rank examinees in the same way as scores based upon a formula in which a penalty is imposed for each wrong answer.[32] Moreover, scoring formulae that penalize examinees for "guessing" assume that all examinees take the same attitude toward a question for which they are not absolutely sure of the correct answer. Such an assumption ignores individual differences among examinees with respect to the personality characteristics influencing risk-taking. A calculated risk by one student may well be considered a wild guess by another. In National Board examinations, examinees are encouraged to answer all questions; no penalty is imposed for wrong answers. The scoring is then based only on the number of questions answered correctly.

Key Validation

National Board examinations are newly created each year to assure that they are current and in step with the rapid advances in medical knowledge. New test items are, however, subject to the hazards of newness. Despite the wise judgment and agreement of panels of experts, the difficulty (P value) or index of discrimination (r_{bis}) of individual items cannot be predicted accurately. A new question may be too difficult or too easy for the examinee population; it may have more than one correct answer that has escaped the closest attention of the examiners; it may contain undetected ambiguities or other technical flaws. Even though the question has been constructed with care, edited diligently and reviewed by several subject-matter experts, the real test of the question is the test of use.

For many practical reasons, among which is the necessity of maintaining the security of the Board's examinations, it has not been considered practical or advisable to pretest items on a selected group of students before an examination is given for purposes of qualification and certification. Until recently, therefore, it has been impossible to keep an examination current by including large numbers of new questions and, at the same time, to pretest the new questions for clarity, appropriateness, difficulty level, discrimination and freedom from technical error.

With the advent of high-speed scoring equipment and computer hardware, it is now possible to obtain an accurate estimate of the performance of each individual test question after the examination has been administered but before final scores are obtained. The process by which this is accomplished has been labeled "key validation." It is a kind of post-test substitute for a pretest. After an examination has been administered, a random sample of examinees is chosen and their answer sheets are scored according to the answer key established by the test committee. Using these scores to establish criterion groups, a full item analysis (see Chapter 4) is performed on the examination. Individual test questions that perform poorly in terms of difficulty and discrimination are identified and reviewed in detail by a psychometric staff member and a medical staff member. On the basis of this review and after consultation with the committee responsible for the test, individual questions performing poorly can be deleted from the examination when the final scoring of the test is done. Thus, it is possible to test each item against the criterion of performance before allowing it to influence the scores of any examinee.

Score Conversion

In an ongoing examination program in which a number of subscores are extracted from each form of the test, it is necessary to provide some mechanism by which scores may be compared from year to year in a particular subject, and from subject to subject within a particular examination. Because examinations may differ in length, item difficulty, and item discrimination, raw scores (number of questions answered correctly) will almost certainly not be comparable from year to year or from subject to subject. Several different approaches are available to convert raw scores to some other scale which will permit comparisons. A simple example is the conversion of raw scores to percentage scores. This operation makes it possible to compare tests of different lengths if one can assume that the tests are similar with respect to other characteristics, such as item difficulty. Unfortunately, however, examinations differ in more ways than simply the number of questions they contain; thus merely converting raw scores to percentage scores is rarely satisfactory.

The conversion system used by the National Board and by many other testing agencies is a linear conversion system; the converted score is derived by applying two constants to the raw score. In its most general form, this system can be expressed by the following equation:

(Eq. 1)

$$Y = a + bX$$

where Y is the converted score
       X is the raw score
       a and b are empirically determined constants

From this equation it is apparent that converted scores can differ widely from each other, depending upon the constants chosen. In fact, the final scale on which converted scores are expressed depends completely upon the manner in which these constants are derived.

One method of determining constants results in what has been labeled "standard scores." Standard scores are used for National Board examinations, for specialty board examinations, aptitude testing and achievement testing programs in many fields. In addition to correcting for differences in test length, standard scores provide a means for correcting for differences in test difficulty and in discrimination level, reflected in the raw score means and raw score standard deviations respectively.

Standard scores are defined as follows:

(Eq. 2)

$$Z = \frac{X - \overline{X}}{SD_x}$$

where Z = standard score
      X = raw score
      $\overline{X}$ = mean raw score of a reference group
    SD_x = raw score standard deviation of the
           reference group

When this basic equation is used, standard scores of the reference group will have a mean of zero, a standard deviation of 1, and, if the distribution of scores is symmetric, half of the standard scores will be negative in sign. In many instances it is more convenient to work with scores with a higher mean (e.g., 500), a larger standard deviation (e.g., 100), and positive signs. These requirements can be met by simply adding appropriate constants to Equation 2 as follows:

(Eq. 3)

$$Z = 100 \left[\frac{X - \overline{X}}{SD_x} \right] + 500$$

Standard scores calculated according to Equation 3 will have a mean of 500 and a standard deviation of 100, regardless of the mean and standard deviation of the raw scores from which they were derived, and will rank examinees in exactly the same way as standard scores obtained using Equation 2.

The equation for converting raw scores to standard scores (Equation 2) may also be expressed as:

(Eq. 4)

$$Z = \left(\frac{-\overline{X}}{SD_x}\right) + \left[\frac{1}{SD_x}(X)\right]$$

Equation 4 then, is Equation 1 in which the a constant is defined as $\frac{-\overline{X}}{SD_x}$ and the b constant as $\frac{1}{SD_x}$. Thus, the equation for converting raw scores to standard scores is a linear conversion equation. Because linear conversions do not alter the order of individual scores, examinees will be ranked in the same way on the basis of their standard scores as they are on the basis of their original raw scores.

A somewhat different linear conversion was used until recently for National Board examinations in order to be able to report passing scores as 75 or higher. Since this had been traditional in days of essay tests, medical schools and students were familiar with this passing level and many state boards of medical licensure had it written into state law. Also from the essay tests, 88 or above was recognized as an honor score. These two points, 75 as the passing level and 88 as the honor level, were two key scores that established the scale upon which this conversion was based. These two scores therefore had the same meaning over time and from test to test. The linear equation from converting raw scores to these "scale scores" (not to be confused with the standard scores described above) was derived by solving the following set of simultaneous equations:

$$U\ (a) + b = 88 \qquad\qquad \text{(Eq. 5)}$$
$$L\ (a) + b = 75 \qquad\qquad \text{(Eq. 6)}$$

where U = the raw score defining "honor" performance

where L = the raw score defining minimum passing performance

Subtracting Equation 6 from Equation 5 yields an equation in one unknown (a) which can be solved. Once the value of a has been determined, this value can be inserted into either Equation 5 or Equation 6 to find the required value of b which will satisfy both equations. The a and b constants derived in this manner are then inserted into Equation 1 and used to convert all raw scores to scale scores. Again, because scale scores are derived from a linear conversion equation, examinees would be ranked in the same order by their scale scores as by their original raw scores.

From the foregoing discussion it is apparent that the conversion process is necessary in the handling of score information to provide the test user with data comparable from test to test and from year to year. It should also be apparent that the conversion process has no necessary relationship to the setting of standards for passing or failing an examination. Standard setting (see pages 62 to 65) is a judgmental process by which a certifying agency defines the lowest level of performance on an examination acceptable for purposes of certification. Score conversion, on the other hand, is a mechanical operation which may be performed on any set of scores, regardless of whether or not a standard is established for the test from which these scores are obtained.

Validity

One of the most important questions asked about any examination is: To what extent does the test measure those characteristics of examinees that the test is intended to measure? The question of test validity always implies some criterion against which the test may be compared. The ultimate criterion for testing the validity of National Board examinations would be the performance of physicians in practice. The actual performance of physicians, with all of its subtleties and variables, is, however, far more complex and hence far more difficult to measure adequately than most of the behavioral criteria developed to date in other occupations. In the absence of ultimate criteria, the validation of tests such as the National Board examinations depends upon the identification of intermediate criteria which can be measured and which appear to be related to performance in practice. A number of such intermediate criteria are available.

In any examination of educational achievement, one of the most important intermediate criteria is the content of the educational system which the test attempts to measure. The test is valid, in this sense, if it measures that which is being taught within the educational system. Because National Board examinations are constructed by panels of medical educators, according to specifications determined by medical educators, the probability that these tests measure what in fact is being taught in the educational system is extremely high. The manner in which the National Board has studied the relevance of Parts I and II has already been described in relation to the criteria and analysis of individual items (see Chapter 4). If individual items can be considered relevant to the objectives of medical education, their content and hence the content of the examination as a whole can be judged as valid. As noted earlier (Chapter 4), National Board questions were considered appropriate for testing current medical education by most of the medical educators asked to judge them.

Medical-school grades constitute another intermediate criterion used to validate the Part I and Part II examinations. In 1964[63] medical-school grades were obtained for sophomore and senior students in 37 U.S. medical schools that could report grades independent of National Board scores.

Correlation coefficients were calculated on a school-by-school basis between these grades and scores obtained on Part I and Part II examinations. Correlation coefficients between overall sophomore-year grades and average score on Part I ranged from .63 to .84, with a mean of .76. For senior students the correlation between overall fourth-year grades and Part II average score ranged from .36 to .80, with a mean of .68.*

A third approach used to validate National Board examinations is to identify groups of individuals at different educational levels who could reasonably be expected to differ in terms of knowledge and clinical skill, and then to compare the test performance of such groups to see if corresponding differences in scores occur. In a recent study of the Part III examination, the test performance of students at the end of the third year in medical school was compared with the performance of individuals near the end of their internship year on the same Part III examination. These groups were chosen on the assumption that interns, on the whole, should exhibit a greater degree of "clinical competence" than third-year students by virtue of the kinds of educational experience (increasing responsibility for patient care) normally occurring during the fourth year in medical school and during the internship. In terms of their Part III average score, 90 per cent of the third-year students fell below the mean of the intern group; differences of similar magnitude were found for each of the subsections of the Part III examination.

An extension of this study, using the same basic procedure for identifying criterion groups, compared the performance of these same junior students with their subsequent performance on an equivalent Part III examination taken after they had completed eight months of their internship training. The results of this longitudinal study were almost identical with the results of the earlier cross-sectional study; the test performance at the internship level was again substantially better than performance as third-year students, with 91 per cent of the third-year scores falling below the mean internship score.

Because, as noted earlier, ultimate criteria of physician performance are not available, it is unlikely that any intermediate criterion will provide the "critical experiment" to confirm or deny unequivocally the validity of National Board examinations. On the other hand, the validation studies that have been done, combined with the judgment of those who create the examinations, provide evidence that the examinations do measure what they are designed to measure.

Reliability

Reliability has been defined in a number of ways, but the most useful definition appears to be one which considers reliability as the capacity of

---

* An earlier study of the correlations between National Board Part II scores and fourth-year cumulative averages of medical-school grades had showed very similar results (see Chapter 4, page 36).

an instrument to provide measures reproducible over time. Instruments used for measuring common physical properties (rulers, scales, thermometers) generally have a high degree of reliability in this sense, so high, in fact, that users of such instruments rarely need to be concerned about this important property of measuring instruments in general. Examinations are a very different kind of instrument and the measurement made by them, i.e., examination scores, are subject to all of the complex factors that produce variability in human behavior. Therefore, tests are not as likely to provide reliable (reproducible) measurements as are instruments that measure simple physical characteristics. Some of the factors influencing behavior (such as learning) are precisely the ones an examination attempts to measure; others (such as the emotional state of the examinee during the test) may produce unwanted variability in examination scores and thus reduce the degree to which the test will yield consistent results. The question of reliability, therefore, assumes major importance in evaluating any testing procedure.

A high degree of reliability alone does not guarantee that an examination will measure that which it is designed to measure. For example, a highly reliable test of medical knowledge might not be appropriate for measuring a physician's attitude toward patients. However, an examination that appears to measure important characteristics but has low reliability may be worse than no examination at all. Such instruments will almost certainly provide misinformation about the characteristics of individual examinees, and may lead to erroneous conclusions about the value of various educational programs if the test performance of groups of examinees is used as a criterion for judging these programs.

Ideally, one would measure the reliability of an examination by administering the test at least twice to a representative group of the examinees for whom the examination was designed and then calculating the correlation coefficient between the scores obtained on the two administrations of the test. However, in addition to the practical problems involved, this approach encounters the potentially serious problem of "practice effect" from the first administration of the test. Individuals may remember test questions from one administration to another and, therefore, the examinee group may be expected to change as a result of the first administration. Their performance on the second administration, then, is a function both of the reliability of the test and the effects of having taken the test once before, and the correlation between their scores on the two testings will probably not provide an accurate estimate of the reliability of the instrument.

An alternative approach to estimating test reliability requires only one administration of the test. In this procedure (split-half technique), the examination is divided into two half tests (e.g. odd-numbered questions assigned to one half and even-numbered questions assigned to the other half); scores are then obtained for each half test and the correlation coefficient between the half tests is calculated.

It has been demonstrated[66] that one of the characteristics of a test having a direct influence upon its reliability is its length. Thus, the final step in calculating reliability with the split-half technique is to estimate the size of the correlation coefficient between the half-test scores (reliability coefficient) for a test twice as long as either of the halves, i.e., for the test as a whole. This is done by applying the following formula (a version of the Spearman-Brown prophecy formula) to the correlation coefficient between the half tests:

$$r_T = \frac{2r_H}{1 + r_H}$$

where r_T = the reliability coefficient
for the test as a whole

where r_H = the correlation coefficient
between the half tests

The split-half method of estimating reliability eliminates the problem of "practice effect." This approach is not entirely satisfactory, however, because there are many ways in which a test may be divided into two halves.* Any method chosen for splitting the test will be somewhat arbitrary, and the resulting reliability coefficient will be slightly different than the one that would have been obtained if a different method of splitting the test had been used.

This dilemma can be resolved when individual item statistics are available for an examination. The reliability of the test can then be estimated so that only one solution is provided and all of the possible interactions between examinees and individual items are taken into consideration. In a sense this technique treats each individual question as a subtest, rather than concentrating on only two of the many half tests that could be considered. A number of investigators[29,37,59] have explored this general approach to estimating test reliability and in 1937 Kuder and Richardson[39] published a series of formulas for calculating test reliability from individual item statistics. One of these formulas has been widely accepted by psychometricians as a substantial improvement over the split-half technique. Known as Kuder-Richardson Formula 20, it is currently used for estimating the reliability of many examinations, including most of the tests prepared by the National Board. It is as follows:

---

* If there are 2N items in a test there are $\dfrac{(2N)!}{2(N)!(N)!}$ ways in which these items may be divided into half tests each of which contains N items. For example, there are 92,378 ways in which a test of 20 items could be split into two half tests of 10 items each.

$$r = \frac{K}{K - 1} \left[\frac{S^2 - \sum_{i=1}^{K} p_i \, q_i}{S^2} \right]$$

where r = the reliability coefficient for
the examination

K = the number of scorable units (items)
in the examination

S = the standard deviation of the test
in raw-score units

p_i = the percentage of examinees answering
the ith question correctly (the P value
for the ith question)

$q_i = 1 - p_i$

Even though the Kuder-Richardson technique differs from the split-half method with respect to the way in which the reliability coefficient is calculated, the K-R 20 coefficient may be considered as a generalized form of split-half reliability such as one might obtain by averaging all of the split-half coefficients that would be obtained if an examination were in fact divided into all possible pairs of half tests and a correlation coefficient calculated for each pair.

Another valuable investigation of the properties of the K-R 20 coefficient was done by Swineford[68] in 1959. She showed that the K-R 20 reliability coefficient can be estimated fairly accurately simply from the number of items in the test and the mean discrimination index (r_{bis}) of those items. Thus, the two major factors determining the reliability of a test are test length (as indicated earlier) and the "quality" of individual test questions in terms of their ability to discriminate between criterion groups of examinees.

All of the indices of reliability cited above are expressed as correlation coefficients with maximum values of 1.00. In interpreting the reliability coefficient, the question arising immediately is a practical one: How large must this correlation coefficient be in order that the test user may have confidence in the testing instrument? While no precise answer can be given, the following guidelines used by the National Board may be helpful:

1. If the reliability coefficient for an examination is less than .70, scores from that test should not be used for evaluation of individuals or groups.

2. If an examination is to be used only for comparing the performance of *groups of individuals* (e.g., mean scores of school classes or groups of physicians) a reliability coefficient of .70 or higher is acceptable.

3. If an examination is to be used to distinguish between *individual examinees* (e.g., candidates for certification), the reliability coefficient should be .90 or higher.

The reliability coefficient for a test is directly related to another statistical property of the examination also of value in judging the accuracy with which the test measures. This statistic is known as the standard error of measurement and is defined as follows:

$$\text{SEM} = S\sqrt{1 - r}$$

where SEM = the standard error of measurement

S = the standard deviation of test scores

r = the reliability coefficient for the test

The standard error of measurement provides a means of determining the range within which the scores of an individual examinee might be expected to vary by chance alone at a specified level of probability if he were tested again with the same examination and if no "practice effect" had occurred as a result of the first test with the same examination.* It should be noted that the size of the SEM (and, therefore, the range within which a score might vary by chance alone) decreases in relation to the square root of the reliability coefficient. Thus, a test with a reliability of .75 yields a SEM of about one-half of a standard deviation unit, whereas a reliability of .90 reduces the SEM to only about one-third of a standard deviation and a reliability of .95 shrinks the SEM still further to less than one-fourth of a standard deviation.

The important aspects of reliability as it pertains to achievement testing may be summarized as follows:

1. A high degree of reliability is a necessary but not sufficient condition for a good examination.
2. The reliability of a test can be estimated accurately from information obtained from a single administration of the test.
3. Reliability is a function of *test length* (number of items) and *quality* (discriminating power) of the individual items within the test.
4. If an examination is to be used for distinguishing between *individual examinees*, a higher degree of reliability is necessary than if the test is to be used only for comparing the performances of *groups*.
5. The precision with which a test measures increases as the square root of the reliability coefficient. Thus, fairly small increments in the reliability coefficient can produce rather large improvements in precision.

* Assuming that an examination with a reliability coefficient of .95 yielded scores having a standard deviation of 5 points, the SEM would be 1.1. The chances are about 2 to 1 that an examinee who obtained a score of 80 on this test would obtain a score between 79 and 81 if he were tested again with the same test.

Establishing Grading Standards

The major purpose for creating any achievement test is to distinguish between individuals who have met some standard of excellence and those who have not. While testing instruments such as National Board examinations may also serve other useful purposes (e.g., providing diagnostic feedback to individual examinees, serving as a yardstick to help measure the effects of curricular change), the basic reason for these tests is to arrive at a decision as to whether an individual can be considered qualified for a license to practice medicine. Therefore, a crucial problem for the examination system is setting a standard for passing or failing the test.

In order to establish a standard, a choice must be made between setting an *absolute* standard of performance or adopting a *relative* standard. An absolute standard is one which requires that examinees answer some predetermined number or percentage of questions correctly to pass the examination. A relative standard, on the other hand, is one in which the pass-fail level is determined by selecting a point on the distribution curve of some group of examinees who have taken the test.

Absolute standards for certification of physicians have great appeal on emotional grounds. One would like to believe that there is some absolutely minimal amount of knowledge, depth of understanding, and degree of skill which every physician must have achieved before he is permitted to practice medicine, even in the confines of a teaching hospital under the close supervision of resident and attending staff. But how much knowledge is enough? To what degree must he understand? Exactly how skillful must he be?

Efforts have been made to set absolute standards for achievement tests in medicine. In grading essay examinations, for example, the examiner frequently has some idea regarding the minimum amount of information that must be supplied by the examinee in order to "pass" an individual question or the examination as a whole.

A method for attempting to set an absolute standard for an objective test, proposed by Nedelsky[56] in 1954, has been used by some medical schools and at least one specialty board.[42] In this procedure a "minimum passing level" (MPL) is determined for each individual test item, these MPLs are summed for all items, and the resulting overall MPL is adjusted by an arbitrarily chosen constant to arrive at the standard for passing the examination. To arrive at an MPL for each item, the examiner must first define a minimally acceptable student and then decide which of the answers to each test question would be recognized as wrong by minimally acceptable students but not by unacceptable students. This procedure appears to be similar to asking the examiner to predict the difficulty level of each individual test question, for a subsample of the examinee group, without benefit of previous performance statistics for the questions. Moreover, if the resulting standards are to be fair to all examinees, examiners must be consistent from subject to subject and from year to year in deciding upon MPLs. Otherwise, standards may fluctuate in an unpredictable fashion and examinees who fail may well have a legitimate complaint about the capriciousness of the certification system.

While the MPL is emotionally appealing, one must question whether examiners can make such predictions with a high degree of reliability and validity, and whether the resulting standards can have the stability required for an instrument that is to be used for purposes of certification.

Attempting to set an absolute standard for examination performance is an extremely difficult task, even when the test is limited to a particular course in a particular medical school taught by the same individual who creates the examination. Therefore, it is not surprising that the medical educators who construct National Board examinations find it impossible to set absolute standards for these tests, which cover fairly broad areas of medical knowledge and will be taken by students with a wide variety of educational experiences.

To provide an illustration of the pitfalls associated with the use of absolute standards for a nationally-administered examination, a retrospective study of the National Board Part I examinations was undertaken. In this study it was assumed that during the two preceding years an absolute standard had been established for each of the six individual basic-science subject tests in Part I and that a student would have been required to answer 60 per cent of the questions correctly to pass each test. Under these conditions, in the first year the average failure rate for one subject would have been about 10 per cent and for another about 20 per cent. In the next year, the failure rates for these two subjects would have been reversed! It would have been difficult, indeed, to explain this degree of variability in failure rates in terms of caliber of students, revised medical-school curricula, or any other reason which would justify holding to this absolute (but quite arbitrary) standard.

The simple fact, reconfirmed by this study, is that the difficulty of examination questions may change unpredictably from subject to subject and from year to year. Absolute standards may not compensate for these fluctuations, and therefore may be unstable criteria for determining eligibility for certification.

A discerning critique of criterion-related measures (absolute standards) in medical education has been given by Dale Mattson, formerly director of the Division of Educational Measurement Research of the Association of American Medical Colleges. He points out: "There can be no question that criterion-related measures have a ready appeal to educators. Examining a person's knowledge, skills, and judgment in relation to a task which he will be required to perform seems to be the only sensible way to attack the problem of assessing competence. By doing so, one eliminates the much maligned 'curve grading' which establishes pass-fail levels on the basis of how classmates have performed. Nevertheless, it is the author's view that criterion-related measures in education are almost universally a delusion and that, in fact, virtually all assessment can be found, under close scrutiny, to be based on performance relative to the performance of a norming group."[49]

Relative standards achieve stability of failure rates from subject to subject and from year to year because these rates are predetermined for some fairly large reference group. For National Board examinations, the reference group is the total group of students taking the examinations as candidates for certification, a constantly increasing number now well over 5,000 students annually. Standards are set so that about 13 per cent of the candidates will fail in each of the basic-science areas and about 4 per cent in each of the clinical areas. This system yields a failure rate of about 10 per cent for the Part I examination as a whole and failure rates of about 2 per cent for Part II and for Part III.

The major argument advanced by critics of relative standards is that the population of examinees upon which the standards are based may change—either suddenly as a result of new and different kinds of individuals introduced into the system, or gradually as a result of evolutionary processes within the system. Therefore, the argument continues, if an examination system imposes a fixed failure rate, individuals who would have failed in the past may now pass the test or vice versa, depending upon the direction in which the examinee population has shifted.

This argument fails to consider a number of important factors that can alter this apparently inevitable conclusion. First, it is unlikely that the competence of the large mass of medical students will show any drastic change, either upward or downward, in a relatively short period of time. Thus, in the short run, when a large percentage of the student population is included in the reference group a relative standard should be at least as stable as an absolute standard.

Second, it appears that in the long run the performance expected of the student is related to the quality of students electing medicine as a career and to the quality of the medical education they receive. Many educators believe that the student of today is better prepared, more highly motivated, and more able intellectually than the student of 20 years ago, and that the medical educational system of today is substantially better than it was in the past. However, the level of expectation, in an absolute sense, also appears to be greater than it was in the past. Many would not now be satisfied with a performance considered minimally acceptable 20 years ago.

In addition, one must consider the effect of an absolute standard upon the educational system itself. If an absolute standard were established, the educational system would undoubtedly attempt to gear its selection mechanisms and teaching programs to meet this standard. In time, and at some cost, any reasonable standard probably would be surpassed by all but a very few individuals, and the failure rate for the certification process would approach zero. As this would occur, the motivational value of certification would diminish and, in the end, the very process which provided a strong incentive for educational change would no longer operate to produce continued improvement in the educational system.

Finally, the use of relative standards does not imply that such standards are fixed for all time. If there is reason to believe that the needs of society have changed, or that the caliber of medical students has changed, the relative standards by which students are judged can and should also be changed. The use of relative standards does not deny the need for judgment on the part of the medical educators who constitute the National Board. Rather, it focuses this judgment on the quality of the individuals being examined and the needs of the society in which these individuals will ultimately function.

CHAPTER 7

Results of Examinations Reported to Medical Schools

Each year the deans and department chairmen of medical schools receive confidential memoranda reporting the performance of their student classes on National Board examinations. Quite obviously these reports apply only to schools in which an appreciable number of students take the examinations. Where a relatively small proportion of a class is included in the examinations, average scores have little value for judging the performance of the class in one major subject in comparison with its performance in other subjects, or for comparing mean scores of the class with mean scores of the national population of National Board candidates or with classes in other medical schools.

A report of the results of the Part II examination for 1971 is included here as an example of the amount and type of information routinely made available to medical school faculties; a similar report is distributed annually for the Part I examination. Another report is prepared for the Part III examination so that medical schools may see how their graduates performed at a clinical level one year after graduation. For all schools receiving these reports, detailed information is made available to indicate how one student class compared with another and with the national averages, in a listing in which the identity of individual schools is meticulously protected. Thus, medical school faculties may judge, on the basis of precise, objective examinations, how well or how poorly their students handled the comprehensive examinations and the several categories for which subscores are reported.

Candidates and Non-candidates

There is a considerable and consistent difference between the performances of candidates (those who elect to register as candidates for ultimate National Board certification, irrespective of whether the examination is a requirement of their medical school) and the non-candidates (students who take the examination only as a requirement of their medical school). The candidates invariably have mean scores higher than those of the non-candidates. Among the factors that may lie behind this difference are the attitudes toward the examinations of both students and faculty. If students are required to take National Board examinations without much forewarning, and are assured that the results will in no way affect their school grades or their standing in their class, they may have little motivation to do well. Knowing that they may derive no personal benefit from them, they may have a casual or even antagonistic attitude toward the examinations. Under these circumstances the results cannot be compared fairly with those in which students are trying to do their best. The results are meaningless and may even be misleading.

In addition to motivational factors, it is likely that some of the difference between candidates and non-candidates is due to a self-selection process. Because the decision to take examinations for National Board credit is largely in the hands of the individual student (even though a school may require him to take the tests), it is reasonable to assume that those students confident of passing are more likely to take the tests for credit than are those less sure of their ability to do well. The less confident students may be tempted to take their chances with state board examinations at a later date. In some schools where Part I or Part II grades count heavily in determining final class grades (i.e., where students are highly motivated), significant differences in test performance still occur between the candidate and non-candidate groups. In this situation it appears that self-selection in the candidate group, rather than motivational factors, explains the difference in performance.

Too Much Reliance on National Boards

Prior to the introduction of multiple-choice techniques in the examinations of the National Board, faculties of medical schools had to rely upon their own assessments of their students' acquisition of medical knowledge. When the results of reliable extramural examinations became available, a new instrument for educational measurement was accessible to the medical faculties. Those who were members of National Board test committees brought to their faculty colleagues an awareness of the objectivity, validity, and reliability of these examinations. Extramural measurements were introduced as comprehensive evaluations of students at periodic points along the four-year course (Part I at the end of the second year and Part II at the end of the fourth year). An increasing number of department chairmen elected to substitute National Board examinations for in-course tests and also for final departmental examinations. The instrument intended to be a useful aid to faculties in judging their students had, in some instances, become the sole determinant of student advancement and even graduation.

The National Board has frequently expressed its disapproval of such use—or misuse—of the results of its examinations but does not consider it appropriate to become involved in the intramural policies of any medical school. Test scores derived from extramural examinations may be useful in appraising student performance, but were never intended to relieve the faculty of its own responsibility in making periodic or final judgments about its students.

Report of a Part II Examination

Following is an example of a report of the Part II examination administered to 6939 fourth-year medical students in the United States in April 1971; an additional 1185 third-year students took the April examination. Great emphasis is placed upon maintaining the confidential nature of the information contained in these annual reports. The performance of the students of each school is made available only to that school and is not released to any other school or agency. With this information in hand the school may, if it wishes, compare its students with the total population of students taking this examination or with students in other schools, but without knowing the identity of any of these other schools.

Table 1 lists the names of the 77 medical schools in the United States in which 25 or more fourth-year students took the Part II examination in 1971. In 58 schools, the examination was taken by at least 90 per cent of the fourth-year students. In 54 schools students were *required* to take the Part II examination either as candidates or non-candidates in April of the third or fourth year. (The tabulations here include only the fourth-year students.)

Scores on National Board examinations are standardized (see Chapter 6) such that the average score for all fourth-year students from the United States and Canada taking the examination as *candidates* is 500; the standard deviation is 100. For the 1971 Part II examination this group totaled 5,877, of which 98.2 per cent received a minimum passing standard score (290) or higher. These statistics are shown in Table 2 together with the average scores and standard deviations for each subject and for the total test for all fourth-year *non-candidates*.

Table 1. U.S. Schools in Which 25 or More Students Took the 1971 Part II Examination

(N = 77)

University of Arizona College of Medicine
Medical College of Alabama
Albany Medical College
Boston University School of Medicine
Bowman Gray School of Medicine of Wake Forest College
University of California School of Medicine, Los Angeles
University of California School of Medicine at San Francisco
Case Western Reserve University School of Medicine
Chicago Medical School
University of Chicago School of Medicine
University of Cincinnati College of Medicine
University of Colorado School of Medicine
Columbia University College of Physicians and Surgeons
Cornell University Medical College
Creighton University School of Medicine
Duke University School of Medicine
Albert Einstein College of Medicine of Yeshiva University
Emory University School of Medicine
Georgetown University School of Medicine
George Washington University School of Medicine
Medical College of Georgia School of Medicine
Hahnemann Medical College
Harvard Medical School
Howard University College of Medicine
University of Illinois, The Abraham Lincoln School of Medicine
Jefferson Medical College
Johns Hopkins University Medical School
University of Kansas School of Medicine
University of Kentucky College of Medicine
Loma Linda University School of Medicine
University of Louisville School of Medicine
Stritch School of Medicine of Loyola University
University of Miami School of Medicine
University of Maryland School of Medicine
Meharry Medical College School of Medicine
University of Michigan Medical School
University of Minnesota Medical School
University of Missouri School of Medicine
Mount Sinai School of Medicine

University of Nebraska College of Medicine
New Jersey College of Medicine
University of New Mexico School of Medicine
New York Medical College
New York University School of Medicine
State University of New York Downstate Medical Center (Brooklyn)
State University of New York at Buffalo School of Medicine
State University of New York Upstate Medical Center (Syracuse)
University of North Carolina School of Medicine
Northwestern University Medical School
University of Oklahoma School of Medicine
University of Oregon Medical School
Medical College of Pennsylvania
University of Pennsylvania School of Medicine
Pennsylvania State University College of Medicine (Hershey)
University of Pittsburgh School of Medicine
University of Rochester School of Medicine and Dentistry
St. Louis University School of Medicine
Medical University of South Carolina
University of Southern California School of Medicine
Stanford University School of Medicine
Temple University School of Medicine
University of Texas Medical Branch (Galveston)
University of Texas Southwestern Medical School at Dallas
Tufts University School of Medicine
Tulane University School of Medicine
University of Utah College of Medicine
Vanderbilt University School of Medicine
University of Vermont College of Medicine
University of Virginia Medical School
Medical College of Virginia
University of Washington School of Medicine
Washington University School of Medicine
Wayne State University School of Medicine
West Virginia University School of Medicine
Medical College of Wisconsin
University of Wisconsin Medical School
Yale University School of Medicine

Table 2. Candidate and Non-candidate Performance on the 1971 Part II Examination (4th-Year Students Only)

CANDIDATES (N = 5,877)

Average standard score for total test and for each subject .   .   .   500
Standard deviation for total test and for each subject   100
Minimum standard score required to pass   290
Per cent pass on total test 98.2

NON-CANDIDATES (N = 1,062)

SUBJECT	AVERAGE STANDARD SCORE	STANDARD DEVIATION
Medicine	424	107
Surgery	430	115
Obstetrics–Gynecology	438	107
Public Health & Preventive Medicine	424	111
Pediatrics	428	110
Psychiatry	425	112
Total Test	407	118

Per cent pass on total test: 85.3

Table 3. Comparison of the Performance of Your Students on the 1971 Part II Examination with the Performance of Students from Other Schools in Which 25 or More Students (Both Candidates and Non-candidates) Were Tested.

School Withheld	Withheld
Number	Name

Number Tested Your School:

Candidates	Total class—number withheld
Non-candidates	None
Total	Total class—number withheld

Percent of your students who passed the total test: 98.1

SUBJECT	AVERAGE YOUR STUDENTS	MEDIAN ALL SCHOOLS	YOUR RANK*	CHANCE RANGE OF YOUR RANK
Medicine	477	479	44.0	31.0–51.0
Surgery	461	482	57.5	50.0–67.0
Obstetrics–Gynecology	492	486	31.0	20.0–42.0
Public Health & Preventive Medicine	453	484	59.5	53.0–67.0
Pediatrics	450	480	67.0	59.0–69.0
Psychiatry	537	484	3.0	3.0– 7.0
Total Test	472	477	46.5	33.0–54.0

* Number of Schools Ranked 77

This report has no references to pass rates for separate subjects of Part II. Since the sole criterion for passing Part II is performance on the complete examination regardless of level of performance on separate subjects, the National Board does not determine or report a pass or fail for individual subject examinations. Examinees are advised that subject scores below 400 may be considered to reflect areas of weakness, i.e., a score of 400 is at about the 15th percentile in the candidate group.

Table 3 applies to one of the schools in Table 1. The name of the school and the number of students are withheld, in keeping with the strict policy of maintaining the confidential nature of the information. The table lists the per cent of the school's students who passed Part II. It also shows, for each subject and for the total examination, the average standard score for the students in this school, the median scores for the 77 schools included in this report, this school's rank among the 77 schools and the range within which the rank-order position of this school could be expected to vary by chance alone ($\pm$ 1 standard error of the average).

Table 4 shows the relative position of all schools with respect to average total grade. The average total grade for each school where Part II is required of all fourth-year students is represented by a W on this chart. Schools that require Part II, but where most students take the test in the third year, are shown as Xs. The average total grade for schools that do not require Part II but in which at least 90 per cent of the students took the examination voluntarily as candidates is represented by a Y. Those schools where less than 90 per cent of the class took the test are shown as Zs. The average total grade for the students in the school selected as this example has been circled. The bracket indicates the range within which this average score might be expected to fall by chance alone ($\pm$ 1 standard error). The solid horizontal line represents the median score of all schools (477).

For each of the six traditional department-oriented subjects that make up Part II, a test committee of medical educators develops an outline of the subject matter and designs the examination to conform to this outline. The subtest has both content validity and a sufficient number of questions to yield a reliable subscore. Other categories of subject matter are, however, derived from a cross-classification of test questions designated according to body system, etiology, or certain special areas (see Table 5). For these categories there has been no outline to assure content validity of a subtest, nor a specified number of questions to assure sufficient content for a reliable subscore. For example, throughout a Part II examination and its 900 to 1000 test questions, cross-classification might identify 80 or 100 questions considered applicable to neoplasm. The number of test questions might then be sufficient for a reliable subscore if the purpose were to compare mean scores of groups. (Higher reliability is required for measurement of individuals.) An appropriate sampling of the knowledge of neoplasm would not be assured, however; a subscore might or might not have validity.

Table 4.   Distribution of Mean Total Grade for 77 U.S. Medical Schools—April, 1971
(fourth-year students)

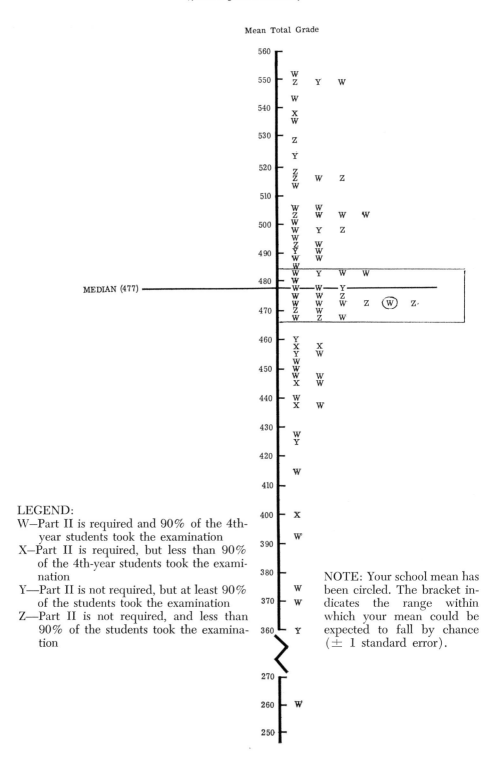

Mean Total Grade

LEGEND:
W—Part II is required and 90% of the 4th-
    year students took the examination
X—Part II is required, but less than 90%
    of the 4th-year students took the exami-
    nation
Y—Part II is not required, but at least 90%
    of the students took the examination
Z—Part II is not required, and less than
    90% of the students took the examina-
    tion

NOTE: Your school mean has
been circled. The bracket indicates the range within
which your mean could be
expected to fall by chance
(± 1 standard error).

Table 5. *Subject-Matter Areas Available for Item Analysis, 1971 Part II.*
(Each area contains at least 25 test items)

DEPARTMENTAL

Medicine
Surgery
Obstetrics and Gynecology
Pediatrics
Preventive Medicine and Public Health
Psychiatry

SYSTEM

Endocrine
Blood
Mental
Nervous
Circulatory
Respiratory
Digestive
Genitourinary
Female Reproductive
Skin and Cells
Musculoskeletal
Special Senses

ETIOLOGY

Immunology
Genetic–Congenital
Infectious
Metabolic–Nutritional
Neoplastic
Behavioral–Emotional
Fluid and Electrolytes
Socioeconomic
Physical–Chemical Agents

SPECIAL AREAS

Newborn
Pregnancy
Biostatistics
Special Preventive Measures
    (Epidemiologic Control)
Radiology
Health Services
Drugs, Therapy and Toxicity
Epidemiology
Growth and Development
Community–Society

If members of a faculty are interested in obtaining detailed information about the performance of their students in any of the cross-classification categories—or in any of the six basic subjects (see Table 5)—a special analysis may be done on request of the department chairman. This analysis shows for each item in the specified category the per cent of the class answering the item correctly in comparison with the per cent of National Board candidates answering the item correctly (i.e., the P value of the class versus the P value of candidates for each item in the category). A confidential copy of the examination is provided with the analysis. A faculty member can then judge the performance of his students in relation to his own opinion of the difficulty and importance of individual test questions. He may, for example, find that his students have shown very little knowledge of a particular question, but he may view the question as relatively unimportant and something that he would not expect his students to know. On the other hand, he might find that 50 per cent of his students missed a point that, in his opinion, they really should have known. In this manner the results of the examination can provide a direct and detailed feedback to a medical-school faculty. Objective data become available for studies of the performance of the class in relation both to the faculty's own concept of curriculum objectives and to the effectiveness of the teaching program in reaching these objectives.

CHAPTER 8

Uniform Standards: National and International

The National Board's collection of test questions, used and calibrated against standards of medical education throughout the United States, provides a resource that is drawn upon as a basis for setting standards for an increasing number of examination programs. Since precise information is available to identify the difficulty of each question and its ability to discriminate between the more competent and the less competent examinees, an examination made up of such questions can be related to standards that are current and sensitive to the dynamic nature of medical education throughout the United States.

Among the groups drawing upon this resource are the Federation of State Medical Boards, the Educational Council for Foreign Medical Graduates, the Medical Council of Canada, and most of the American specialty boards.

Federation Licensing Examination (FLEX)

The Background for FLEX. Despite early misgivings about the institution of a "national" qualifying examination and its relationship to the legally constituted licensing authorities of the states,[11,65] the state boards themselves came to recognize the advantages and superior quality of the National Board's multiple-choice examinations. In 1953, soon after the Board's change-over from essay examinations, Connecticut was the first state to request the National Board to provide examinations to be administered under state law in place of essay examinations prepared and graded by its own Board of Examiners. The move was well received. The state board had an external criterion, i.e., the performance of medical students and graduates throughout the United States, against which to judge the performance of its own candidates, many of whom were graduates of foreign medical schools. The idea spread to other states, especially those with large numbers of candidates; New York, Massachusetts, Virginia, and Illinois soon followed Connecticut's lead.

Over the course of several years, an increasing number of states elected to take this route to a higher quality of licensing examination. Concurrently the Federation of State Medical Boards sought, through a series of examination institutes, to achieve greater uniformity of standards for medical licensure while, at the same time, preserving the constitutional right of each state to regulate and control the practice of medicine within its borders. In 1967, the Federation's Examination Institute Committee, expressing an earnest desire to move constructively toward its declared objective of uniform standards for determining qualification for a medical license, sought the assistance of the National Board. By this time the Board was providing approximately 25,000 tests annually for 16 state boards for the examination of about 3000 physicians. The trend was well established.

These two developments—the increasing use of test questions derived from the National Board's standardized pool of material and the determination of the Federation's Examination Institute Committee to achieve a higher quality of state-board examinations—led to an agreement between the National Board and the Federation for the development of a Federation Licensing Examination (FLEX), the objective of which was to place state medical licensing examinations and procedures in definite relationship to modern medical education with special emphasis upon the clinical competence of candidates for a state license.

The Examination. A test committee of members representing those state boards participating in or interested in adopting the FLEX examination meets regularly with the staff of the National Board to design and to construct the examination. The members of this committee, all of whom are representatives of state boards, are responsible for selecting the questions according to their collective judgment as to the appropriateness of each item for candidates for a state license. As the committee members know from experience in their own states, many of these candidates have graduated from medical school many years earlier; many of them will have had backgrounds with widely differing standards and curricula; and many may be unfamiliar with much that is to be found in the current pool of National

Board test material, especially in the basic medical sciences. The committee, therefore, gives careful attention to the relevance of each question for the current practice of medicine.

The examination extends over three days. The first day includes the six traditional basic medical science areas, providing 90 test items in each subject. The basic-science subjects are: anatomy, biochemistry, microbiology, pathology, pharmacology, and physiology. The items are arranged in interdisciplinary form so that the subject-matter origin of an individual item is not identified for the candidate. The second day includes the six traditional clinical-science areas, also with 90 test items in each subject. The clinical-science subjects are: internal medicine, obstetrics and gynecology, pediatrics, preventive medicine and public health, psychiatry and surgery, including items in medical jurisprudence. These items, too, are presented in interdisciplinary form.

The third day of the test contains test material drawn from the National Board's Part III examination. It includes clinical material presented in the form of pictures of patients, gross and microscopic specimens, roentgenograms, electrocardiograms, charts and tables, about which searching questions are asked. A distinctive feature of the third day is the programmed testing based upon patient management problems, to assess the candidate's judgment in the sequential management of clinical problems similar to those encountered in day-to-day practice (see Chapter 5).

The scoring of the FLEX examination is done by the National Board and is related directly to the performance of National Board candidates as determined by the item analysis of the test questions. Since the difficulty of each item (the P value) and the index of discrimination (r_{bis}) are known for each item, an accurate estimate may be made of the scores that would be expected for National Board candidates if they were to take the FLEX examination.

Although each of the three sections of the examination is set up and presented to the candidates in interdisciplinary form, without identification of its component subjects (i.e., as a scrambled examination), a score is derived for each major subject in order to satisfy state laws and regulations. Many states require numeric scores in specified subjects, most often in terms of 75 per cent for a minimum passing level. (One wonders about the origin of the 75 per cent level, and even more about the meaning of 75 per cent of the knowledge of a subject such as internal medicine. The only possible explanation is that this minimal level is traditional. At any rate, the tradition persists to the extent that the FLEX examination scores are reported so that a scale score of 75 can be accepted by state boards as a legally authorized minimum passing level.)

The first step in scoring FLEX is to obtain scores for each of the six subjects of the basic medical science section (Day 1), each of the six clinical subjects (Day 2), and for the clinical competence section (Day 3). The six subject scores for Day 1 are then averaged to give a comprehensive score for the basic medical sciences. Similarly, the six subject scores for the second day are averaged to provide a comprehensive score for the clinical sciences. A weighted average is then determined so as to give major emphasis to clinical competence. The scoring formula gives the basic-science section (the first day) a weight of one, the clinical-science section (the second day) a weight of two, and the test of clinical competence (the third day) a weight of three. This weighted average is reported to the Federation together with the scores on individual subjects and average scores for the basic medical sciences, the six clinical subjects, and clinical competence. The Federation in turn transmits these scores to the individual states. Although each state has the right to interpret the scores in accordance with its own laws and regulations, the FLEX weighted average has become the final determinant of passing or failing in most states, irrespective of the scores on individual subjects and independent also of the one-day averages for basic sciences, clinical subjects, or clinical competence. Thus the scoring method adopted by the FLEX Committee acknowledges the responsibility of state licensing boards in determining the qualification of physicians who have graduated from medical school, who have had supervised responsibility for the care of patients in a hospital as interns or residents, and who may have had additional years of clinical experience before registering for the FLEX examination.

During the first few years of the FLEX program, the failure rate, based upon the weighted average, was approximately 8 to 10 per cent for graduates of medical schools in the United States and approximately 65 per cent for graduates of foreign medical schools.[54]

FLEX and Interstate Reciprocity. Now that the FLEX program has become established and gives every promise of being adopted by most if not all states, it appears altogether likely that those few states choosing to remain outside of this program will encounter more and more difficulty in maintaining interstate reciprocity. In a report, *FLEX Projections for 1969*, presented by Doctors Montgomery and Merchant at the annual meeting of the Examination Institute of the Federation of State Medical Boards in February 1969, the following prediction, the importance of which would be difficult to overestimate, was made: "Those states using a modern technique and uniform baseline will look askance at those states still utilizing an archaic procedure. Endorsement for those non-participating states will become an increasingly serious and unreconcilable problem."[55]

FLEX and the National Board Examinations: A Dual Examination System. A point that continues to need clarification is the relationship between National Board examinations and the Federation Licensing Examinations. The examiners of the National Board (the members of its several test committees) are charged with the responsibility of formulating examinations to test the knowledge of students as they are learning medicine in medical school today. This objective is different from that of evaluating competence to practice medicine for individuals who may be far removed from their formal courses in areas such as biochemistry or anatomy. Since the objectives are different, the examinations should be different—each aimed at its own clearly defined target.

Thus, an entirely logical dual system has developed: the National Board examinations focused upon the student of today who is the physician of tomorrow, and the FLEX examination to assess the basic knowledge and more especially the clinical competence of the physician of today who was the student of earlier years.

Examinations for the Medical Council of Canada

Closely related to the use of the National Board's collection of examination material for FLEX and licensure examinations in the United States is a similar use of this collection of pretested standardized questions for the Medical Council of Canada and official licensure in Canada. Here again a multidisciplinary committee appointed by the Council meets with the medical and psychometric staff of the National Board to formulate an examination according to specifications drawn up by the Council and in keeping with medical education in Canada. These examinations, containing multiple-choice questions in clinical areas and patient management problems, are very like the National Board's Part II and Part III examinations. An additional feature of this program is a translation into French for this bilingual nation. This examination is, then, a logical and sensible step leading to uniform standards of licensure in the United States and Canada, countries having schools accredited on the basis of the same standards and which, accordingly, should have like standards for admission to the practice of medicine.

The ECFMG Examination

Another testing program depending upon the National Board's pool of standardized, pretested multiple-choice questions is that of the Educational Council for Foreign Medical Graduates (ECFMG). This program was initiated in 1958 for the primary purpose of determining, on an individual basis, whether a graduate of a medical school outside of the United States or Canada could be considered sufficiently well qualified to serve as intern or resident in an American hospital, to assume supervised responsibility for the care and well-being of patients, and to profit from an opportunity for graduate medical education in the United States. Before this time, the American Medical Association with the cooperation of the Association of American Medical Colleges had published a list of foreign schools, the graduates of which could be considered on an equal basis with graduates of medical schools in the United States. It soon became apparent, however, that the point of real concern was not so much the caliber of the school from which the individual had graduated as the caliber of the individual himself.

Accordingly, agreement was reached to establish a testing procedure to permit direct comparison between the medical knowledge of any graduate of any recognized medical school in the world* and that of graduates of medical schools in the United States. To achieve this objective the ECFMG turned to the National Board of Medical Examiners and its large collection of questions, for each of which the level of difficulty and index of discrimination were known from previous testing of American students. By appropriate selection and scoring procedures, examinations were prepared so that, if a graduate of a United States school who had taken the National Board Part II examination were to take the ECFMG examination, he would be expected to obtain the same score on the ECFMG examination that he had obtained on the National Board examination.

The ECFMG examinations are all in the English language; it would be impossible to translate them into the many languages of those taking the examination. Furthermore, the basic purpose of the examination is to determine an individual's qualification for an appointment in an American hospital, where he will have to communicate with American physicians and American patients in English. Consequently, a test of the physician's comprehension of spoken English is included in the examination. This English test, although relatively short (taking only about 45 minutes of the testing day), has been found to be a helpful although admittedly coarse screening procedure for determining proficiency in the English language. The test is scored separately. To be considered as having passed the ECFMG examination, a candidate must achieve a passing score on the English test, independent of his score on the rest of the ECFMG examination.†

A score of 75 on the ECFMG examination is passing, and may be said to be equivalent to a passing score on Part II of the National Board examinations. It must not be assumed, however, that passing the ECFMG examination means the same as passing National Board examinations. To achieve certification by the National Board, a candidate must successfully complete a total of five days of examination. The ECFMG examination is completed in one day and, on this one day, 6½ hours are allowed for the number of questions that would have had an allowance of 4½ hours on National Boards. Questions previously used in National Board examinations are carefully selected with emphasis on those elements of medical knowledge generally accepted on a worldwide basis. The essential purpose of the ECFMG examination is to serve as a test of qualification for appointment as an intern in an American hospital, working under supervision. Certification by the National Board, on the other hand, is regarded as a qualification for license for the independent practice of medicine.

During the first thirteen years of the ECFMG program (1958 through

* "A recognized medical school" was defined as any medical school listed in the Directory of Medical Schools published by the World Health Organization.[71]

† Paul R. Kelley, Jr., Ph.D., Associate Director of the National Board of Medical Examiners, deserves special credit for initiating and maintaining the effectiveness of the ECFMG English Test.

1970), 215,757 examinations were administered to graduates of foreign medical schools in testing centers distributed throughout the United States and around the world. During this period, 127,550 individuals were tested. The difference between the number of examinations administered and the number of individuals tested (i.e., 88,207) represents examinations taken by candidates repeating the test, having previously failed on one or more occasions to obtain a passing mark. Since the ECFMG permits individuals to register for the examination as often as they wish, some persistent souls have repeated and failed the examination ten or more times—rather convincing evidence of the reliability of the examination.

Of those taking the ECFMG examination during the first thirteen years, the failure rate averaged approximately 60 per cent. Since, as noted earlier, the standard for passing the ECFMG examination is pegged to the standard of the National Board Part II examination, and since the failure rate for National Board candidates on Part II is consistently about 2 per cent, it may be said that, if National Board candidates at the point of graduation from medical school were to take the ECFMG examination, about 2 per cent would be expected to fail.

Further details concerning the ECFMG examination, including requirements for admission to the examination, broad descriptions of its content, and a record of performance of ECFMG examinees over the years, may be found in the Annual Report of the ECFMG and in the annual medical licensure issue of the *Journal of the American Medical Association.*

CHAPTER 9 ▪ *Examinations as a Guide to Learning*

During medical school a student undergoes a variety of episodic examination procedures designed to determine his qualification for a course grade, for promotion to the next class, or for graduation and an M.D. degree. These may be faculty-made examinations or the extramural examinations of the National Board. At the graduate level he must take and pass examinations of the specialty board in his chosen field if he wishes to be certified as a specialist. All of these examinations have one feature in common: that of determining individual competence or qualification at a specific point in preparation for a career in medicine. This common feature identifies examinations as qualifying examinations, measuring the product of the educational system.

Examinations also serve as guides to learning during the course of the learning process, and therefore become part of the learning process. Careful analysis of examination results provides specific information to the educator relative to teaching, and to the educatee relative to learning. Two examples of such examinations are the "Minitest" at the undergraduate level and in-training examinations for residents at the graduate level. The former provides evaluation of the educational process by measurement of group performance; the latter provide assessments of the achievement of individuals.

The Minitest

The manner in which the results of the National Board's comprehensive examinations are reported to medical school faculties and the uses of these reports in evaluating the effectiveness of the educational process have been described in Chapter 7. The rapidly evolving changes in the medical-school curriculum have resulted in recognition of the need for other means of evaluating the impact and effectiveness of these innovations in the educational process. To meet this need, the National Board has introduced an examination of reasonable length to provide a means of "tracking" the learning process in medical school on a year-by-year basis. A one-day multiple-choice examination was developed which is essentially a miniature Part I and Part II; it has become popularly known as the Minitest.[43]

This method of curriculum evaluation was first introduced by the University of Rochester School of Medicine in 1964, as reported by Hilliard Jason.[38] Its objectives were to provide "a testing instrument that would (a) reliably and validly sample the subject matter content of the four medical school years; (b) contain items which could be depended upon to discriminate effectively among students at a wide range of levels of learning; (c) be of a form which would permit the design of different but equivalent examinations each year in order to make possible repetitive testing of the same students; (d) provide data that could be meaningfully compared to an external norm, which would serve as a base line."

The Minitest consists of 360 pretested questions drawn from all of the major subjects of Parts I and II. A new but equivalent form of the test is created each year. All forms are matched in terms of medical content, based upon category outlines as designated by the basic-science and clinical-science test committees of the National Board. Additional comparability from year to year is maintained by matching the various forms of the test in terms of difficulty and reliability.

The examination is administered at the end of each academic year to all four classes and, in order to obtain a base line for the first-year class, it is also administered to each entering freshman class in early September.

Several schools have undertaken this evaluation program with the administration of the test to all four classes simultaneously. Others have initiated the study with the entering freshman class and have then involved one additional class each year so that, by the end of five years, the program includes all four classes.

The Minitest provides each of the participating schools with comparable information year by year and class by class. Mean performance based on standard scores is calculated for the total test, the basic-science subtest, and the clinical subtest. In addition, further subscores on the subtests in the basic medical sciences are derived for the traditional first-year subjects (a combined score on anatomy, biochemistry, and physiology) and for the traditional second-year subjects (microbiology, pathology, and pharmacology). The latter scores are of particular interest with respect to the first- and second-year students.

Since the questions have been pretested in a regular Part I and Part II examination, each school can compare the performance of its students on the basic-science and clinical portions of the test with the expected performance of National Board candidates.

While this horizontal assessment of the five educational levels—the entering freshmen and each of the four classes at the end of the academic year—is of interest and may give a preview of things to come, it is the longitudinal data accumulated by a given school, year by year and class by class, that should provide useful information about patterns of learning in medical education. At what levels of the educational process do students show significant gains in knowledge of basic science? Is this knowledge further enhanced, maintained, or diminished as students progress through medical school? When do students begin to acquire knowledge of clinical medicine? What is the slope of this curve over time?

As these longitudinal data accumulate in tracking the learning process before and after curriculum change, a medical school can evaluate the effects of new educational programs in relation to patterns of learning.

Evaluation of Learning at the Graduate Level

Whereas evaluation of learning as just described is an operating concept at the medical-school level, little or no attention to such ongoing evaluation procedures is given at the graduate level. To be sure, the program director and others on the staff can and do evaluate the competence and skill of the resident in the day-to-day exchange in the clinic, at the bedside, and in the conference room. Because of its nature, however, graduate education as conducted in a clinical setting poses certain limitations with respect to evaluation of learning.

Since graduate medical education is primarily patient oriented, there is great variation in clinical experience among residents within a given training program. Conferences providing opportunities for evaluation of learning may not be presented in systematic and sequential fashion, since these sessions tend to be patient oriented as well.

Learning at the graduate level is characteristically independent. As the resident assumes increasing responsibility for patient care and also for his own continuing education, the program director has less and less opportunity to observe and to evaluate the progress and learning that may or may not have taken place.

Also, since in most residency programs the resident rotates through related disciplines, the program director cannot always assess the effectiveness of these experiences. He must sometimes depend upon the judgment of those outside the specialty for evaluation of trainee learning.

As a result of these educational variables, all of which limit the evaluation process, basic deficiencies in the learning of the individual trainee may go undetected during the training period.

Following residency training, one or more years of practice experience may be required before a physician is eligible for certification by a specialty board. Such practice experience is relatively unstructured and, therefore, allows for wide variations in the type and quality of learning that may take place. Many years may elapse between the time a physician embarks upon his graduate training and the "moment of truth" when he is confronted by the examination of his specialty board. This examination, intended primarily as a qualifying examination, can come too late in his career to provide a useful learning experience.

One of the most disturbing aspects of the training and certifying procedure in graduate medical education is the high failure rates for those who have completed approved training programs extending over five to seven years and have met all the requirements for the examination. The failure rate may be as high as 40 to 50 per cent.

Since all candidates have been trained in approved programs, have been considered qualified by their respective program directors, and have met all eligibility requirements, these high failure rates are indeed difficult to understand. It would, of course, be naive to assume that all approved programs are of comparable quality, or that individuals entering these training programs are of comparable caliber. Even in the face of these variations in quality, however, why are so many individuals so poorly prepared by the time they reach the certifying examination? What factors account for these failure rates? Is the certifying examination itself at fault? Is the quantity or the quality of graduate training deficient? Do program directors accept and approve trainees who are inadequate in caliber or poorly suited to the specialty concerned?

In-Training Examination for Residents as a Guide to Learning

Seriously concerned about the high percentage of presumably carefully selected and well-trained candidates who failed to pass its qualifying examination after seven or more years of training, the American Board of Neurological Surgery undertook to study its educational programs and qualifying examination.[21,34,44,45,48,57] In 1962, the Board appointed a Commission under the auspices of the American Association of Neurological Surgeons (the Harvey Cushing Society) to study the problem.[34] The objective was to develop a program to improve the quality and effectiveness of residency training in neurosurgery as well as the preparation of individual candidates for certification, and hence to increase the competence of all those entering the specialty.

Various measures were considered. The possibility of giving an aptitude test at the end of the year of internship, before accepting a trainee for specialty training, seemed unrealistic and of questionable value. The possibility of encouraging each program director to conduct an examination of his own every year or two during the training period was considered to have merit, but variable and impractical to implement.

The possibility of conducting a uniform examination during the period of formal training seemed to be theoretically most desirable and likely to provide useful information about both the caliber of the trainee and the quality of the training program. More specifically, the introduction of an in-training examination could, it was hoped, identify areas of weakness in the knowledge of the trainee or deficiencies in the training program itself, so that trainees and their program directors could then endeavor to correct these weaknesses during the course of the training period.

The Commission and the officers of the Board of Neurological Surgery met with the staff of the National Board. Many aspects of the plan were discussed, the objectives of the program were reviewed, and an outline of an examination was drawn up to meet the stated objectives. A multiple-choice examination was developed to measure knowledge and comprehension of those areas of neurosurgery considered to be essential to the specialty: neuroanatomy, neurophysiology, neuropathology, neuroradiology, clinical neurology, general surgery, and neurosurgery proper. To provide sufficient test content to assure the reliability of five specified subscores, the examination called for 500 questions and a total time allowance of six hours.

At the outset, the Commission had intended to offer the examination to residents completing the residency training within two years. It was felt that this would allow adequate time for additional study to correct any areas of weakness disclosed by the examination. Any individual who had already completed his formal training and who wished to take the examination would be allowed to do so, however. In fact, individuals who had previously failed the certifying examination (an entirely oral examination) were encouraged to take the in-training examinations to gain further information about their continuing educational needs.

From the beginning of this program, both the Commission and the Board of Neurological Surgery had emphasized that the examination should be regarded as an in-training evaluation for the purposes of identifying weaknesses in a trainee's preparation and in the training program. Throughout the planning and implementation of the study, all concerned held firmly to the view that the individual results should neither be published nor revealed to the Board. A trainee's performance on the in-training examination could not, therefore, be used at a later date to influence his acceptance for the final certifying examination, nor could it be used by the specialty board to influence the decision as to whether he passed or failed the final examination.

Accordingly, it was decided that a trainee's score for the examination as a whole and his subscores on the component categories would be made available only to the chairman of the Commission, and through him to the trainee himself and to the director of his training program. Thus, only the trainee and his program director would have the opportunity of discussing the scores.

The first in-training examination in neurosurgery was administered in 1964. Completely new examinations, but comparable in content, were developed and administered annually thereafer, and residents had the opportunity to take repeat examinations during the period of their training.

No passing level was applied to the examinations. Each examinee received a report of his score for the total examination and for each of five subtests. He also received frequency distributions in such detail that he could compare his performance with residents at his own level of training, or at more advanced or less advanced levels, referring to designated subcategories of subject matter. Thus, a candidate might find himself deficient in neuroradiology but better than average in other categories of the test. He and his program director could then take appropriate steps to strengthen his knowledge of neuroradiology.

As the program proceeded, impartial and reliable data derived from the examinations served to fulfill the primary objectives set forth by the Commission: to provide direction for learning, leading to improvement in the competence of candidates for Board certification, and also to provide a means for the objective evaluation of individual training programs.

Guy Odom has commented upon the first years of experience with this program:[57] "It is my impression that the in-training written examination also has proved to be highly valuable to the trainee and to the program directors, and there is no question that the examination has decreased the failure rate on the oral examination."

Other specialty societies that have sought the assistance of the National Board in developing examinations for the specific purpose of aiding the learning of the resident are the American College of Obstetrics and Gynecology and the American Neurological Association. As in the case of Neurological Surgery, the National Board works with committees of the specialty societies responsible for the definition, design, and content of the examinations. These examinations consist of 400 to 500 multiple-choice questions and are scheduled to be completed within one day. Subscores are derived in four or five of the major subject-matter categories. Scores for individual examinees are obtained for each subcategory and for the examination as a whole. The scores, with frequency distributions based upon levels of training similar to those distributions for the neurosurgery examinations, provide detailed information for the resident to assess his own areas of relative strength or weakness.

CHAPTER 10 ▪ *Self-Assessment for Continuing Medical Education*

Multiple-choice testing methods, now having gained wide recognition for accurate measurement of medical knowledge, are being applied increasingly to a different and yet closely related phase of medical education usually referred to as continuing medical education.

Traditionally, continuing medical education has been available through assiduous reading of professional journals and through periodic attendance at medical meetings and participation in postgraduate courses offered by medical schools, hospitals and specialty societies. In 1966 a program sponsored by the American Medical Association and known as the Utah Pilot Study undertook to determine, together with other information, the physician's perception of his own educational needs. This information was then to serve as a basis for structuring the content of postgraduate courses.[7,67] A questionnaire was distributed to physicians throughout the state asking them to indicate those areas of medical knowledge in which they felt deficient; in a sense, the physician was asked to specify what he did not know. Obviously the program left much to be desired. If an individual had not even heard of some recent and perhaps important advance in medical knowledge, how could he possibly indicate this in responding to the questionnaire?

A different approach was initiated by the American College of Physicians in 1967.[4,62] The objective was much the same: to provide an opportunity for the physician to identify for himself any gaps in his knowledge so that he could then take steps to educate himself in those areas in which he had found himself deficient. The method, however, was different and far more realistic: It provided the physician with a comprehensive set of multiple-choice test questions which he could study confidentially on his own time, testing his own knowledge of the major areas of internal medicine.

To implement the program, Hugh Butt, formerly chairman of the College's Committee on Educational Activities, requested the National Board to assist in an innovative project that became known as the Medical Knowledge Self-Assessment Program. Sets of multiple-choice questions were formulated by nine specially appointed committees of the College. Each committee consisted of about six individuals and was responsible for one of nine major areas of internal medicine: hematology, pulmonary disease, endocrinology and metabolism, renal disease and electrolytes, rheumatology, infectious disease and allergy, gastroenterology, cardiology, and neurology. To provide adequate coverage of each of the special areas, approximately 80 multiple-choice questions were agreed upon as the goal for each committee. The total set of questions, therefore, amounted to 720.

The committee members formulated questions according to an outline of subject matter they themselves had devised. They then met with the medical and technical staff of the National Board, at which time the questions were accepted, revised or discarded. Emphasis was placed upon current knowledge and concepts, with special attention to new advances applicable to the practice of medicine.

The author of each question was requested to cite one or more references; these were later assembled as a bibliography and sent to each member participating in the program with a report indicating the questions he had answered correctly and incorrectly. The hope and expectation were that he would study the references for each question he had answered incorrectly, and thus would fill in the gaps in his knowledge.

As reported by Edward C. Rosenow, Jr., Executive Vice President of the College:[61] "We think it is extremely newsworthy that almost 9,000 physicians volunteered to take such a self-appraisal without any coercion of any type. We also feel that it is strong evidence that physicians are conscientious about their knowledge and try very hard to keep up." Many letters received by the College were laudatory. The following quotes were cited as typical: "It is the best postgraduate course I have taken in 15 years. I have never been so stimulated." And, "I don't know that it did much for my pride. Nevertheless, the experience was enjoyable, exhilarating and humiliating. Many questions have sent me back to the drawing board."

Here then was a new enterprise applying the experience and technical know-how of designing examinations for precise measurements of individuals and groups to a new mode of continuing education. This form of self-assessment or self-learning was soon emulated by the American Academy of Pediatrics, the American Psychiatric Association, and the American Society of Anesthesiologists. The American College of Physicians launched a second repeat program with a completely new set of questions, and the American College of Surgeons and the American College of Obstetrics and Gynecology have also sought the help of the National Board in developing self-assessment test questions for their memberships. The American Psychiatric Association, the American Academy of Pediatrics and the American Society of Anesthesiologists may soon be expected to repeat the construction of new sets of questions for distribution to their memberships. This form of continuing medical education now appears well established under the sponsorship of the specialty societies.

Initially, the American College of Physicians had intended their program to serve not only as a self-assessment for the individual members of the College but also as an instrument to yield group scores in categories of subject matter.[4] The group scores would then be a valuable guide to the design of the College's postgraduate courses. Emphasis would shift from a course scheduled because the lecturer had a subject he particularly liked to a course focused upon an area of internal medicine in which practicing physicians (those who had participated in the self-assessment program) had demonstrated lack of knowledge.

As the design of the first self-assessment program advanced, however, it was agreed that for the first pioneering venture there would be no attempt to collect either individual or group scores. In order that there would be no doubt whatsoever about absolute anonymity of those registering for the program, no information was sought about areas of special interest, specialty board certification or years since graduation from medical school. Furthermore, there was no uniform procedure for the self-testing exercise. Some participants might wish to consult textbook references, or colleagues, before making their choice for the right answer; others might choose their answers solely from their knowledge of the subject, without recourse to references. For this reason, also, it was clear that scores would be meaningless.

By the time of the American College of Physicians' second program, it was apparent that the membership had lost any apprehension—if ever they had any—that this was some devious plan to obtain covert information about individuals. It was therefore agreed for the second program to obtain confidential information about board certification, areas of special interest, year of graduation from medical school and sources of help (if any) in answering the test questions. Again, assurance was given that the handling of records (through a bonded agency) would ensure that there was no possibility of identifying the answer papers of individual participating physicians. However, the coded biographical data, together with the answers to the question about consulting references, would permit individual participants to learn how well they had answered the questions in comparison with others. For example, a general internist who answered the questions without consulting references could compare his performance with that of other general internists who *said* that they had done likewise. A hematologist could compare his answers to the questions with those of others who indicated subspecialty interest in hematology and who *said* that they had not consulted textbooks or journals.

These scores admittedly lacked the rigor and the reliability of the hardline qualifying National Board or specialty board examinations, conducted under controlled circumstances, simultaneously, in many centers across the country. Nevertheless, this additional feature of providing scores and "norms" for purposes of comparisons was received favorably by the College. One of its primary objectives had now been met: It had obtained reasonably reliable information that could serve to direct its postgraduate courses to meet demonstrated needs.

As more and more attention is paid to self-assessment programs, one of the incentives that prompted them is voiced sometimes openly and sometimes by indirection in low key. Reference is frequently made to the 1966 report of the Citizen's Commission on Graduate Medical Education known as the Millis Commission.[23] This Commission emphasized the need not only for continuing medical education but also for repeated examinations leading to periodic recertification and updating of medical licenses. Since medical licenses are awarded by governmental agencies, the threat of governmental intervention was loud and clear.

Hugh Carmichael, Director of the Office of Continuing Education for Psychiatrists of the American Psychiatric Association, speaks of the viewpoint of his organization as follows: "The attitude and position of the American Psychiatric Association on this question is that we have an antipathy to compulsory measures, which no doubt some of you share, and we hope to forestall their imposition by the success of our program in motivating our members to remedy the serious gaps in knowledge and skills disclosed by our Psychiatric Knowledge and Skills Self-Assessment program by continuing their own self-education."[5]

Self-evaluation programs earnestly undertaken by medical specialty societies for the benefit of their members are substantial contributions to the goals of continuing medical education. They therefore are strong answers to pressures from the public for assurance that a physician, having once been certified as competent, continues to be competent and to keep abreast of recent advances in his field of specialization. It is doubtful, however, that these programs in themselves will fully satisfy this growing demand. Those who accept the invitation to participate in them are apt to be the physicians who take any available opportunity to keep up with current medical knowledge, who come to the meetings of their professional societies and take postgraduate courses. What about those who do not regularly attend medical meetings and are not to be found at postgraduate courses? It is the age-old question so familiar to the clergy: how to get to the fellow who does not come to church?

Assurance as to the competence of the physician is a function of the specialty boards. Two specialty boards, the American Board of Family Practice and the American Board of Internal Medicine, have announced that recertification will be required at periodic intervals. This move, having been started, is likely to gain momentum rapidly. It therefore seems reasonable to predict that even more impetus will be given to self-assessment programs as a means of affording physicians an opportunity to prepare for recertification. It also seems both likely and appropriate that the division of responsibility between specialty societies and specialty boards will continue as it has begun, with the specialty societies extending their efforts in continuing education for their members and the specialty boards seeking to devise and apply more realistic assessments of clinical knowledge and competence for physicians perhaps well advanced in their professional careers.

Oral examinations, as a means of determining the qualification of a physician for the practice of his profession, can be traced back in medical history to at least the twelfth century, when members of the faculty of the University of Salerno met with representatives of the emperor to determine the proficiency of the candidate.[72] The oral (viva voce) examination has continued to this day as a dominant feature of the system for determining whether the years of education, clinical training, and experience of an individual physician have qualified him to undertake the responsibility for the health and often the lives of patients. As licensing and certifying systems evolved, the oral examination sometimes stood alone as the sole determinant of the physician's legal right to practice the profession for which he had spent years in preparation, e.g., the Staatsexamen of Germany. Sometimes the oral examination was preceded by or coupled with written examinations, as in the British Commonwealth.

When the examinations of the National Board of Medical Examiners were first instituted in 1916, and until the oral examination was superseded by more objective methods of assessing clinical competence as described in Chapter 5, the interviews between a candidate and a series of examiners were the principal feature of the National Board's Part III examination, the final step an individual had to take to be judged by the Board as qualified for a license to practice medicine on his own.

Certification as a specialist, in distinction to qualification for a license granted by a state, has developed in the United States as a function of independent specialty boards. Because of the freedom of these boards to establish standards for their own examinations, it is not surprising that wide variations are found in quality, form and content. One board may depend entirely on oral examinations, another may rely upon written examinations with no oral examination. Most specialty boards have a combination of written and oral examinations, the written examination serving as a preliminary screening device. Those who clear the hurdle of the written examination are admitted to the oral examination for the final step leading to certification.

When the oral examination is preceded by a comprehensive exploration of the candidate's knowledge of a specialty, the examiner can—but not always does—assume that the candidate, having passed the written examination, has adequate knowledge of the subject. The time available for the oral can then be spent in assessing attributes and qualifications of the candidate that cannot be measured in a written examination.

The essential feature of the oral examination as conducted formerly by the National Board and as usually conducted by specialty boards is a face-to-face interview between examiner and examinee. A wide variety of adjunctive elements may be used in questioning the candidate. Laboratory specimens, roentgenograms or lantern slides may serve as a basis for discussion of clinical problems. A candidate may be required to obtain a clinical history and do a physical examination on a patient, and then be questioned by the examiner. Did he hear a significant heart murmur and can he recognize its significance? Did he feel the tip of an enlarged spleen or detect an enlarged lymph node?

Edithe Levit, in considering methods of evaluation at the graduate level, has pointed out that they may be classified in two broad categories: examination and observation.[46] Evaluation by means of an objective written examination is concerned primarily with the cognitive educational objectives (knowledge, comprehension, analysis, synthesis) that are quantitative and can be measured precisely. Levit suggests that such evaluation be viewed as in vitro. Evaluation by observation is concerned with behavioral aspects of learning, clinical judgment, technical skill, assumption of responsibility, doctor-patient relationship. These educational objectives are appraised subjectively by means of direct observation, communication, experience and intuition. Such evaluations may be considered as being conducted in vivo, that is, at the bedside, in the operating room and in the laboratory.

When the number of individuals to be examined is small, evaluation by direct observation of performance may be feasible and preferred by the examiner. In the first examination of the National Board, conducted in

1917, there were 10 candidates. (Current National Board examinations may accommodate 6000 to 7000 candidates simultaneously in many examining centers.) Practical demonstrations were principal features of the examination. (To demonstrate his surgical skill, a candidate was required to perform a gastroenterostomy on postmortem specimens from a dog. When he had completed his surgical procedure, the esophagus was connected to a water faucet. If there was no leakage, the candidate "passed" this portion of the examination; this was a practical in vivo evaluation for the candidate, if not for the dog.)

As the numbers of candidates for certifying examinations have increased, practical problems in scheduling and conducting the oral examination have become almost insurmountable, especially when thousands of candidates must be accommodated annually. Examiners are brought from far and near in sufficient numbers to meet the demands of the schedule for a session that may last several days for them, although for an individual candidate the amount of examining time may be only a few hours. If patients are involved as test subjects, hospital services are disrupted—to say nothing of the equanimity of the patients. Some specialty boards with large numbers of candidates call upon their foremost members to contribute amounts of time that appear to be reaching the limit of tolerance. The monetary value of the time contributed by the examiners is beyond calculation, and even the actual costs of travel and accommodations for examinees and examiners are formidable.

In spite of its drawbacks, however, the oral examination is deeply rooted in professional qualifying examinations. The face-to-face interview, the manner and content of the reply to a direct question, the opportunity for the examiner to ask the examinee to clarify or justify his answer, the facility of communication (often judged as an indication of facility of communication with a patient), the direct observation of the attitude and personality of the examinee—all are features of the oral examination that cannot be captured by any form of written examination. Furthermore, the conviction of the experienced examiner that he can recognize quality and competence when he sees and hears them weighs heavily in the balance whenever the value of the oral examination is being considered.

Reliance upon the widely accepted and time-honored oral examination is, however, being widely challenged for purposes of certification at the professional level.[13,20,51,58] Examiners and examining boards appear to be increasingly aware that examinations are a form of measurement and, like other forms of measurement, are subject to tests of accuracy. When the reliability of the oral examination is studied, it almost invariably fails to equal the reliability that can be demonstrated for good multiple-choice examinations.

One of the techniques used to determine the reliability—or lack of reliability—of the oral examination is the inter-rater correlation, that is, the degree to which one examiner agrees with another in judging and grading the same examinee. The principle is logical and similar to the determination of reliability for written multiple-choice examinations when scores on one half of the examination are correlated with scores on the other half (see pages 57 to 59).

Reports of "high reliability" of the oral examination may, however, be misleading when based upon inter-rater correlations. If an examinee is interviewed by two examiners simultaneously, both examiners hear the responses to the same questions, both examiners have the same basis upon which to judge the knowledge, attitude and behavior of the examinee, but neither can avoid being influenced by the reactions of the other, subtle and unspoken though these may be. Under these circumstances the likelihood of a high inter-rater agreement is built into the procedure, and therefore claims for high reliability have little meaning. The situation is comparable to claims of high reliability for a multiple-choice examination based upon agreement resulting from two passes of an answer sheet through a scoring machine.

A case in point is the report of Carter[6] following an analysis of data from the oral examination of 250 candidates for certification by the American Board of Anesthesiology. Examiners worked in pairs, interviewing the same candidate in the same room. Under these conditions the agreement between examiners was found to be "very good" (average of the correlations was .62). Based in part on this observation, Carter concludes that these oral examinations can be highly reliable. This conclusion is questionable. As noted earlier (see page 61), the reliability of an examination that is to be used to distinguish between individual candidates should have a reliability coefficient of .90 or higher.

If, on the other hand, a single examiner or group of examiners interviews an examinee and the score resulting from this interview is then compared with that from another interview by another examiner or group of examiners, a more realistic appraisal of the inter-rater situation can be made. For example, some years ago Hartog[27] tested the degree of consistency of two individual groups of examiners in interviewing the same examinees under carefully controlled circumstances. He came to the conclusion that it was largely a matter of chance whether the combined judgment of the one group was in agreement with that of the second.

When, in 1960, the National Board undertook to study and to develop objective methods of evaluating the clinical competence of physicians, the new techniques resulting from this study and described in Chapter 5 were looked upon as possible supplements to, rather than substitutes for, the traditional bedside examination. An attempt was made to improve the reliability of the bedside examination with a carefully devised evaluation form (see page 43). This method was used over a three-year period as a part of the examination, but a study of the correlation between the independent evaluation of the two examiners for a single candidate showed that the agreement was still only at the chance level ($r = 0.25$ for a total of 10,000 examinations).[35] The bedside "practical," oral examination was therefore discontinued by the National Board in 1963.

An extensive study of the certifying examinations has been undertaken and reported as a collaborative program of the American Board of Orthopaedic Surgery and the Center for the Study of Medical Education of the University of Illinois.[24,40,41,51,52,53] In addition to extensive revision of the written examination, the oral examination was completely redesigned to reduce the variables and increase the reliability of this portion of the certifying assessment. Examiners were diligently prepared to make uniform evaluations of the candidates, and standardized materials were coupled with weighting scales specifying the aspects of performance to be judged by the examiners. Also, in an attempt to eliminate the variable introduced by patients as testing subjects, the examiner plays the role of a patient and the examinee elicits a history that has been preformed and is the basis of the examination. This innovative procedure, even with built-in attempts to standardize it, does not avoid the hazard of subjective judgment although it appears to measure a skill somewhat different from those measured by paper-and-pencil tests (communication with patient). Its reliability as reported by Levine and McGuire[41] is below that which would be considered acceptable by the National Board for a certifying examination.

Others concerned with the certification of physicians for general or specialty practice have followed much the same route: (1) seeking to improve the reliability and effectiveness of the oral examination, thereby preserving the features which all agree are important and which cannot be accomplished in a written examination or (2) using or developing other measures of professional competence with at least some, if not all, of the desirable features of the oral examination and, at the same time, demonstrable reliability.[8]

An American specialty board faced with very large numbers of candidates to be examined annually, the American Board of Internal Medicine, has critically analyzed its oral examination. It was concluded that the oral examination for certification in general internal medicine should be discontinued, and that emphasis should be placed upon objective measures of professional competence similar to those of the National Board's Part III examination.[1]

Some years ago, in a world-encompassing view of examinations, John R. Ellis[15] presented an illuminating, succinct and informal estimate of oral examinations from his point of vantage as General Secretary of the Association for the Study of Medical Education, London, and Dean of the London Hospital Medical College:

> In Britain, irrespective of the number of written tests, and whether essay type or (as is increasingly common) objective type questions are used, by far the greatest weight is placed upon bedside, clinical, interview examinations. This remains the case, despite all sorts of practical

difficulties, such as finding suitable patients, gathering them together in sufficient quantity for increasingly large numbers of candidates, and keeping the whole enterprise in action for several days on end.

A strange aura surrounds these examinations in clinical subjects. Traditionally known as "finals," they have dominated the lives of the candidates for the three years of their clinical study. They have been the ultimate goal. Yet, in most schools, and particularly in those in which the examinations are external, the students have no clear concept of what is expected of them, or of what constitutes, as it were, the syllabus of knowledge, skills, attitudes, and methods of thought upon which they are going to be tested. In general, they take their guide from the dim past, leaning heavily on what their predecessors—either immediate or as remote as their fathers—have told them.

The candidates believe that the clinical tests count most—in which respect they are at one with the examiners; that they will be expected to give a correct diagnostic label to each of the patients—in which respect they differ from many, but not all, of their examiners; that it will help to wear a dark suit, a clean collar, and a meaningful tie and to, somehow, exhibit a demeanor in which respectful subservience to the examiner is combined with one of great independence of thought and yet a marked sense of responsibility. This, I think, occasions great problems for the increased number of female candidates, who obviously must choose the kind of hairdo, dress, and jewelry which will attract the male examiner, and yet not be thought likely to distract the patient. At interview tests in some schools, academic gowns are worn; in Galway the girls appear in elbow length gloves.

Finally, students are convinced that luck plays a large part in deciding the issue. Charms are secreted on the person, and astute beggars who position themselves near the entrance do extremely well. Luck does, undoubtedly, play a large part; luck in getting or spotting eight questions out of the whole of medicine about which one can show some knowledge; luck in getting an easy case in the clinical, or a patient who states clearly what is wrong and what is right; luck in getting an examiner who is neither more nor less intelligent than oneself, one who is feeling friendly, and who is prepared and able to put his questions clearly; luck in having obtained enough marks in medicine to persuade the obstetricians at the joint examiners' meeting to give one more mark, so that with passes in obstetrics and medicine, the surgeons may be prepared to raise their mark by two, thus providing a pass in all three subjects.

This situation (and I do not think that I have described it unfairly) sounds unsatisfactory. It is perfectly true that in, for example, what is called the long case in medicine—when the candidate, in the space of about one hour, takes a history, makes an examination, and discusses his findings with two examiners—they are going to judge a whole series of different variables. These must include: clinical technique; factual knowledge; attitudes; personality; and the abilities to recall arrangements of data, recognize syndromes, interpret information, and solve problems.

These factors are seldom, if ever, tested separately or assessed separately, and if concentration upon one thing at a time is of any value, then these examinations are unlikely to prove much more than a sort of rough and ready assessment. Yet there is a strong belief (amounting almost to a faith), that the English clinical, conducted by two examiners, of whom one at least is highly experienced in the art, is sufficiently accurate for the purpose, and that many of the dimensions which are assessed cannot be assessed better in any other way. This deeply felt belief is, I think it must be admitted, largely untouched by knowledge of what other techniques might be used or are being used elsewhere. It has its origins, perhaps, and some justification, in the fact that clinicians are more accustomed than others, and therefore probably better than others in making important decisions on inadequate data.

In Britain, we do not talk merely about good examinations; we talk also about good examiners. We say, "Oh, so-and-so? I can't say that I like the man, but I must say he is a good examiner," in the same way that we might say he is a good horseman. I suppose that in the United States examiners are ceasing to exist; in a way, it is rather sad, because there is something romantic about them—like the cavalry, and other things that have had to go with the changes in the times.

CHAPTER 12 ▪ *A Computer-Based System for Evaluation of Clinical Competence*

As the oral examination has been subjected more and more to questions and criticisms such as those mentioned in the preceding chapter, it has become a matter of compelling importance to find better ways of evaluating the competence of the physician. The question is basic: Is this individual, after years of education in medical school and supervised clinical experience in a hospital, qualified to assume general or specialized responsibility for the care of patients?

The *knowledge* of the physician-candidate can be measured in whatever degree of breadth and depth is deemed appropriate by his examiner. In written examinations, the candidate can be challenged both to assemble his facts and to apply them to the solution of the problem in hand. Knowledge, as the foundation for clinical judgment, can be measured with precision. The evaluation of *judgment* as an essential component of clinical competence is more elusive.

The National Board of Medical Examiners in its Part III examination has had many years of experience with objective methods of measuring clinical competence, and has assisted specialty boards in introducing similar methods into their certifying examinations; these methods, however, although representing significant advances in test technology, are not good enough. Better ways are needed to answer the basic question as to whether the physician-in-training has reached the point were he can emerge from this training qualified for a license to practice medicine or for a certificate as a specialist.

Furthermore, both the public and the profession are voicing doubts about the once-and-forever certification of the specialist. As pointed out earlier, the principle of periodic evaluation and recertification, possibly at intervals of about six years, has been openly espoused by at least two specialty boards. Other boards are considering such action. Here then is another urgent reason for development of more sophisticated methods of measuring the clinical competence of physicians who may be well advanced in their professional careers and who may have become highly specialized. Testing procedures that are effective at the time of initial licensure or certification may not fill the need for evaluation for those whose experience has been in a limited area.

In its constant and continuing search to measure ever more precisely both the process and the product of medical education, the National Board undertook to explore the feasibility and the practicability of computer technology for objective evaluation of clinical competence. Instruction in which the computer assumes the function of teacher or textbook had become well established. It seemed reasonable to assume that the computer might be programmed to play the role of examiner or patient, or both.

A Prototype CBX

A long-range research program was initiated with the financial support of the Carnegie Corporation and The Commonwealth Fund. A pilot project resulted in a prototype for a computer-based examination (CBX), developed as a cooperative project with the Laboratory of Computer Science at the Massachusetts General Hospital and the Department of Continuing Medical Education of the Harvard Medical School.[36]

In this prototype examination, the examinee sits at a computer terminal (see Fig. 1). He holds in his hand a small booklet given to him as he registers for the examination. This booklet lists in a general index all the questions about the patient that the computer is programmed to answer— on history, physical findings, laboratory tests and diagnostic procedures.

The examinee must first gather all pertinent information about the patient by asking questions related to the clinical history and physical examination. From the general index he selects the questions he wishes to ask. He then enters the numbers of these questions in the computer terminal. The computer responds immediately. For example, if the physician should ask about the patient's weight, the patient (computer) might reply: "I have lost some weight recently." A second question about weight might

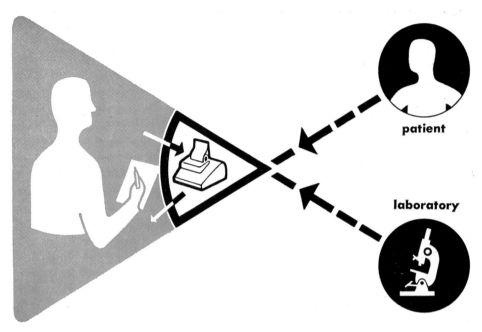

FIG. 1.

be asked with the further response: "I have lost forty pounds in the last year." The physician-examinee proceeds in this manner to ask other questions he considers directly related to the patient's problem. The responses printed out by the computer then provide a record of the clinical history and physical examination.

Because several different clinical skills are being measured by the CBX, the test in this initial prototype model is such that the examinee's responses in the history, physical examination, differential diagnosis, and laboratory sections are evaluated separately. At the end of each stage in the management of the patient's problem, all information that should have been obtained during that stage is given in summary form. After the examinee has obtained a clinical history, the computer will provide any additional essential information that he will need as a base line for reliable measurement of his competence in handling the next stage of the clinical problem. He then proceeds to find out about the physical findings he thinks would be particularly helpful in the light of what he has learned from the history.

Following a review of the summary of the history and physical findings printed out by the computer, the examinee then formulates a differential diagnosis. He again refers to the index for a general listing of diagnoses. He selects those he considers highly probable and enters them by number in the computer. Then he is given a list of all diagnoses that should have been included in the differential diagnosis, and is again brought to the same base line and confronted with the same problems in the further assessment of his use of diagnostic studies and procedures.

The next step provides the examinee with a simulated opportunity to use a large hospital laboratory and the services of special departments. In the general index he finds a listing of all laboratory studies and other procedures that the various diagnostic facilities programmed in the computer can perform. The situation is similar to that in a hospital or clinic where the physician must consult a laboratory manual listing the studies the laboratory will perform. If he considers it important to determine blood glucose, the computer might print out "90 mg per 100 ml." If he wishes a roentgenogram of the chest, the computer will print out the report as it would come to him directly from the radiology department. Although the results are given specifically, the index of questions and procedures is purposely so generalized that the physician must first determine in his own mind the questions he considers pertinent to the patient's problem and the laboratory procedures and diagnostic studies he wishes to order.

After the results of the requested diagnostic studies have been reported by the computer in response to specific requests, the final diagnosis is called for. The program might then challenge the examinee to support his diagnosis, drawing upon the information he has gathered about the patient, and thus simulating one of the features of many oral examinations. The computer-based examination may end at this point or it may continue in a sequential step-by-step manner to follow the patient's course for days, weeks or months.

At every step of the examination, the computer has a record of the information that the examinee has requested from the patient and from the diagnostic facilities. Since each entry in the general index has been identified as a correct or incorrect decision at that point in time, scores can be derived from the questions the examinee has asked (or failed to ask) in taking the history, the diagnostic studies he ordered (or failed to order) and his competence in arriving at a diagnosis and plan of management. Several different methods of scoring and evaluating the interaction between physician and simulated patient are being investigated.

Special Features of the CBX

Many features of the computer-based examination in clinical competence distinguish it from its paper-and-pencil ancestor. It simulates the patient and clinical setting more realistically than has been possible in any paper-and-pencil test. Of special importance is the fact that it requires the examinee to initiate his own decisions and avoids the cues inherent in multiple-choice tests, where the examinee has a limited number of choices from which he must select those he considers correct. Further, the story is locked in the computer, so that the examinee cannot decide what to do on the first day of hospitalization by reading ahead to the patient's condition on the second day. Also, this method of testing makes it possible to track the sequence of the examinee's decisions and to alter the responses and scoring.

For example, if the physician should order a protein-bound iodine determination and an intravenous pyelogram, the PBI level would depend upon the sequence of the studies; the scoring would be adjusted accordingly.

Another use of the computer with an interesting potential in evaluating the clinical competence of the physician is its capacity to recalculate moment by moment the probability of various diagnoses based upon all data accumulated to that point in the management of the patient. A new status of the simulated patient then may emerge from the simultaneous solution of linear and differential equations relating physiological parameters.[64] Used thus, the computer would do more than file and return data; it would provide entirely new ways to assess aspects of a physician's ability to manage situations similar to the real and practical problems of patients.

Practical Applicability of the CBX

The unique features of the CBX offer great promise for qualifying examinations, especially at the graduate level. This promise must, however, be tested through further research and development before it can be proved a reliable instrument to discriminate between the adequately and the inadequately qualified candidates for a medical license or for specialty-board certification. Furthermore, assuming that the validity and reliability of a computer-based examination can be fully established, examining a single physician at a single computer terminal is quite different from examining 500 or 5000 examinees at the same time in many locations across the country. The problem then becomes that of establishing a nationwide network of computer facilities with multiple terminals at designated centers, all operating simultaneously. However, the rapid advances in network facilities and telecommunications systems suggest that the network problem can be solved and will be solved by the time the method has been adequately tested and established. Unquestionably, the CBX will go through many generations before it meets the strict criteria of reliability and validity as an instrument for objective evaluation of clinical competence. Also, it seems clear that the development of such a system, with its more precise definition of competence and a network of communication facilities, will be of as much value in medical education as it will in testing.

Bibliography

1. American Board of Internal Medicine: Written (certifying) examination in internal medicine. Bull. Amer. Coll. Physicians, 12:236, 1971.
2. Anastasi, A.: *Psychological Testing*, 3rd ed. The Macmillan Company, New York, 1968.
3. Bloom, B. S.: *Taxonomy of Educational Objectives: The Classification of Educational Goals*. David McKay, New York, 1956.
4. Butt, H. R.: Medical knowledge self-assessment program. Bull. Amer. Coll. Physicians, September 1967.
5. Carmichael, H. T.: Self-assessment tests: The psychiatric knowledge and skills self-assessment program. JAMA, 213:1656, 1970.
6. Carter, H. D.: How reliable are good oral examinations? Calif. J. Med. Res., 13: 147, 1962.
7. Castle, C. H., and Storey, P. B.: Physicians' needs and interests in continuing medical education. JAMA, 206:611, 1968.
8. Corley, J. B.: Examinations of the College of Family Physicians of Canada. Personal communication.
9. Cowles, J. T., and Hubbard, J. P.: A comparative study of essay and objective examinations for medical students. J. Med. Educ., 29:14, 1952.
10. Cowles, J. T., and Hubbard, J. P.: Validity and reliability of the new objective tests. J. Med. Educ., 29:30, 1954.
11. Derbyshire, R. C.: *Medical Licensure and Discipline in the United States*. The Johns Hopkins Press, Baltimore, 1969.
12. *Directory of Medical Specialists*, Vol. 14. Marquis, Chicago, 1969.

13. Ebel, R. L.: *Essentials of Educational Measurement*. Prentice-Hall, Englewood, in press.

14. Ebel, R. L.: Ability versus knowledge in testing educational achievement. National Board Examiner, Vol. 16, 1969.

15. Ellis, J. R.: Examinations abroad. Proceedings of Conference Commemorating the 50th Anniversary of the National Board of Medical Examiners, 1965.

16. Fan, Chung-teh: Item analysis table. Educational Testing Service, Princeton, 1952.

17. Fitzpatrick, R., et al.: *Development of Objective Flight Checks and Proficiency Measures for Use with Bomber, Reconnaissance and Cargo Crews*. American Institute of Research, Pittsburgh, 1954.

18. Flanagan, J. C.: The critical requirements approach to educational objectives. School and Society, 71:321, 1950.

19. Flexner, A.: Medical education in the United States and Canada. Bulletin #4, Carnegie Foundation for the Advancement of Teaching, New York, 1910.

20. Foster, J. T., Abrahamson, S., Lass, S., Girard, M. A., and Garris, R.: An analysis of an oral examination used in specialty board certification. J. Med. Educ., 44: 951, 1966.

21. Furlow, L. T.: Report of the study commission of the American Board of Neurological Surgery. J. Neurosurg., 27:381, 1967.

22. Gordon, T.: The development of a standard flight check for the airline transport rating based on the critical requirements of the airline pilot's job. Report 85, Civil Aeronautics Administration, Washington, 1949.

23. *The Graduate Education of Physicians*. American Medical Association, Chicago, 1966.

24. Gregory, C. F.: Orthopaedics and the impact of the learning theory. J. Med. Educ., 44:777, 1967.

25. Guilford, J. P.: *Fundamental Statistics in Psychology and Education*, 3rd ed. McGraw-Hill, New York, 1956.

26. Gulliksen, H.: *Theory of Mental Tests*. John Wiley and Sons, New York, 1950.

27. Hartog, Sir Philip, and Rhodes, E. C.: A viva voce (interview) examination. In *The Marks of Examiners*. The Macmillan Company, London, 1936.

28. Hickam, J. B., Deiss, W. P., and Frayser, R.: Intramural use of extramural examinations. JAMA, 192:830, 1965.

29. Hoyt, C.: Test reliability estimated by analysis of variance. Psychometrica, 6: 153, 1941.

30. Hubbard, J. P.: The role of examining boards in medical education and in qualification for clinical practice. J. Med. Educ., 36:94, 1961.

31. Hubbard, J. P.: Programmed testing in medicine. In *Testing Problems in Perspective* (Anastasi, A., Ed.). American Council of Education, Washington, 1966.

32. Hubbard, J. P., and Clemans, W. V.: *Multiple-Choice Examinations in Medicine*. Lea & Febiger, Philadelphia, 1961.

33. Hubbard, J. P., and Cowles, J. T.: A comparative study of student performance in medical schools using National Board examinations. J. Med. Educ., 29:30, 1954.

34. Hubbard, J. P., Furlow, L. T., and Matson, D. D.: An in-training examination for residents as a guide to learning. New Eng. J. Med., 276:448, 1967.

35. Hubbard, J. P., Levit, E. J., Schumacher, C. F., and Schnabel, T. G.: An objective evaluation of clinical competence. New Eng. J. Med., 272:1321, 1965.

36. Hubbard, J. P., Levit, E. J., Barnett, G. O., Goldfinger, S. E., Dineen, J. J., Farquhar, B. B., Schumacher, C. F.: Computer-based evaluation of clinical competence. Bull. Amer. Coll. Physicians, October 1970.

37. Jackson, R. W. B.: Reliability of mental tests. Brit. J. Psychol., 29:267, 1939.

38. Jason, H.: Sequential examinations in assessing the impact of a new medical curriculum. J. Med. Educ., 41:18, 1966.

39. Kuder, G. R., and Richardson, M. W.: The theory of estimation of test reliability. Psychometrica, 2:151, 1937.

40. Levine, H. G., and McGuire, C.: Role-playing as an evaluative technique. J. Educ. Meas., 5:1, 1968.

41. Levine, H. G., and McGuire, C.: The validity and reliability of oral examinations in assessing cognitive skills in medicine. J. Educ. Meas., 7:63, 1970.
42. Levine, H. G., and McGuire, C.: Use of profile system for scoring and reporting certifying examinations in orthopedic surgery. J. Med. Educ., 46:78, 1971.
43. Levit, E. J.: Use of the National Board "Minitest" for evaluation of curriculum change. J. Med. Educ., 42:930, 1967.
44. Levit, E. J.: Comments regarding further study of graduate training in neurosurgery. J. Neurosurg., 27:385, 1967.
45. Levit, E. J.: Evaluation of learning. Arch. Derm., 99:343, 1969.
46. Levit, E. J.: Evaluation of learning in graduate education. J. Neurosurg., 30:348, 1969.
47. Lindquist, E. F. (Ed.): Educational Measurement. American Council on Education, Washington, 1951.
48. Matson, D. D.: An in-training evaluation of residency training programs and trainees. J. Med. Educ., 41:47, 1966.
49. Mattson, D. E.: Criterion-related measures in education. J. Med. Educ., 46:185, 1971.
50. McGuire, C.: A process approach to the construction and analysis of medical examinations. J. Med. Educ., 38:556, 1963.
51. McGuire, C.: The oral examination as an assessment of professional competence. J. Med. Educ., 41:274, 1966.
52. Miller, G. E.: The orthopaedic training study. JAMA, 206:601, 1968.
53. Miller, G. E.: The study of medical education. Brit. J. Med. Educ., 3:51, 1969.
54. Montgomery, L. G.: Recommendations and opinions of the Examination Institute Committee. Fed. Bull., 57:359, 1970.
55. Montgomery, L. G., and Merchant, F. T.: FLEX, projections 1969. Fed. Bull., 56:266, 1969.
56. Nedelsky, L.: Absolute grading standards for objective tests. Educ. Psychol. Meas., 14:3, 1954.
57. Odom, G. L.: Neurological surgery and the assessment of accomplishment. J. Med. Educ., 44:784, 1969.
58. Pokorny, A. D., and Frazier, S. H., Jr.: An evaluation of oral examinations. J. Med. Educ., 41:28, 1966.
59. Richardson, M. W., and Kuder, F.: The calculation of test-reliability coefficients based upon the method of rational equivalence. J. Educ. Psychol., 30:681, 1939.
60. Rimoldi, H. J. A.: Rationale and application of tests of diagnostic skills. J. Med. Educ., 38:364, 1963.
61. Rosenow, E. C., Jr.: The medical knowledge self-assessment program. Bull. Amer. Coll. Physicians, August 1968.
62. Rosenow, E. C., Jr.: The medical knowledge self-assessment program. J. Med. Educ., 44:706, 1969.
63. Schumacher, C. F., and Kelley, P. R., Jr.: Correlation between medical school grades and scores on examinations of the National Board of Medical Examiners. Unpublished report.
64. Senior, J. R.: Personal communication.
65. Shryock, R. H.: Medical Licensing in America, 1650–1965. The Johns Hopkins Press, Baltimore, 1967.
66. Spearman, C.: Coefficient of correlation calculated from faulty data. Brit. J. Psychol., 3:271, 1910.
67. Storey, P. B., and Castle, C. H.: Continuing Medical Education. American Medical Association, Chicago, 1968.
68. Swineford, F.: Some relations between test scores and item statistics. J. Educ. Psychol., 50:26, 1959.
69. Thorndike, R. L. (Ed.): Educational Measurement. American Council on Education, Washington, 1971.
70. Watson, C. J.: Some activities and impacts of the American Board of Internal Medicine. JAMA, 138:257, 1948.
71. World Health Organization: Directory of Medical Schools, Geneva, 1963.
72. Womack, N. A.: The evolution of the National Board of Medical Examiners. JAMA, 192:817, 1965.

Test Questions Used in Examinations of the National Board of Medical Examiners

The following test questions are examples of those used in National Board examinations, and have been drawn from the Board's collection of calibrated test questions (pool) described in Chapters 1 and 3. Each of the types (forms) of multiple-choice questions in current use is represented by one or more examples.

One hundred questions have been selected from the six traditional basic medical sciences (Part I): anatomy, biochemistry, microbiology, pathology, pharmacology, and physiology; 100 from the six clinical subjects (Part II): internal medicine, obstetrics and gynecology, pediatrics, preventive medicine and public health, psychiatry, and surgery. Additional questions used and tested in the Part III examination illustrate the use of pictorial material in each of the three parts of the National Board's examinations. A set of patient management problems demonstrates the special feature of the Part III examination familiarly known as PMP (see Chapter 5).

(The set of 100 questions in the basic medical sciences and that in the clinical subjects are not to be mistaken for a full Part I or Part II examination. A test of 100 multiple-choice questions would normally take 1½ hours.

Both Part I and Part II consist of 800 to 1000 test questions and are scheduled for a total of 12 hours.)

Based upon the item analysis derived from the use of these questions for National Board candidates, the difficulty of the abbreviated sample "test," expressed as the average number of times each item was answered correctly by the candidates and spoken of as the mean P value (see page 32), and the effectiveness of the test in discriminating the high-scoring from the low-scoring group of candidates, referred to as the r index (see page 33), have been calculated for each set of 100 items.

	Mean P value	Mean r index
100 Basic Science Questions	.68	.37
100 Clinical Questions	.67	.35

The difficulty level of each of these two sample tests is approximately that of National Board examinations, where the mean P value is usually in the range of .60 to .65. The mean r index for these two sets of questions, .37 and .35, respectively, is somewhat higher than that expected for a complete Part I or Part II examination because, in these sample tests, only questions that have performed well when used have been selected, whereas the full Part I and Part II examinations are newly constructed each year and therefore contain test questions not yet put to the test of usage.

The few examples of pictorial material are taken from a section of the Part III examination that would usually contain approximately 120 test questions scheduled for a 2½-hour examination. These examples, however, are sufficient to give some impression of the versatility of this testing method in contrast to the "slide quiz" familiar to several of the American specialty boards, where the candidate has a few predetermined seconds or minutes to view one picture at a time as projected on a screen; he cannot compare one picture with another as when, for example, a series of blood smears is printed in the test booklet as the basis for a differential diagnosis or when, as demonstrated in these samples, a series of electrocardiograms is the basis for several questions.

The set of patient management problems (PMP) related to a single patient demonstrates the testing method forming the main part of the single day scheduled for Part III. In the actual examination, the candidate would encounter 10 or 12 such sets for a testing session of 3½ or 4 hours. Since this testing technique is less familiar than that of multiple-choice questions, carefully worded and detailed instructions are printed on the cover of the test book and time is allowed for the examinees to study these instructions carefully.

When the PMP test is printed for use in an examination, a block of erasable ink is printed over each response to hide the information given for the result of a selected choice of action. The examinee must then remove this ink with an ordinary hard eraser to reveal the result of his decision. (For purposes of this demonstration, the responses have been screened to indicate the erasable ink blocks.) To obtain a fair impression of the task involved in taking this test, the reader should endeavor to look *only* at the response for the single choice of action he has selected before making the next choice and looking at the next response.

In the instructions preceding the test, candidates are informed that, in scoring these problems, they are given credit for correct choices and are penalized for errors of commission (selection of incorrect courses of action) and omission (failure to select correct courses of action).

When the PMP included here was used in a Part III examination, the average National Board candidate made 30 correct choices and five incorrect choices. The remaining ten choices were accorded a zero score, neither correct nor incorrect, as indicated in the answer key. These responses are included to round out a realistic medical situation, but are either of equivocal importance or represent actions which might or might not be appropriate or "correct" in a particular medical center.

Part I—Examples of Questions Drawn From Basic Science Subjects: Questions 1–100

DIRECTIONS: Each of the questions or incomplete statements below is followed by five suggested answers or completions. Select the one that is BEST in each case.

1. Which of the following veins is a part of a portal system?

    (A) Right ovarian
    (B) Left ovarian
    (C) Middle rectal
    (D) Superior rectal
    (E) Uterine

2. Sinusoids interposed between two sets of veins are found in the

    (A) small intestine
    (B) spleen
    (C) anterior pituitary gland
    (D) placenta
    (E) parathyroid glands

3. The edema of acute inflammation involves the exudation of protein-rich fluid

      (A) primarily through venules and capillaries
      (B) primarily through arterioles
      (C) only through capillaries
      (D) through lymphatic vessels
      (E) through all microvessels more or less equally

4. A factor responsible for edema in the nephrotic syndrome is

      (A) increased filtration pressure of the blood plasma
      (B) decreased osmotic pressure of the blood plasma
      (C) decreased capillary permeability
      (D) retention of potassium
      (E) increased blood lipids

5. Carbon dioxide is transported in the blood primarily as

      (A) dissolved CO_2
      (B) carbonic acid
      (C) carbaminohemoglobin
      (D) plasma bicarbonate
      (E) intracellular bicarbonate in red blood cells

6. The release of carbon dioxide from blood in pulmonary capillaries is retarded by

      (A) the simultaneous absorption of oxygen
      (B) any increase in the alveolar carbon-dioxide tension
      (C) carbonic anhydrase
      (D) the chloride shift
      (E) the buffer effect of hemoglobin

7. A molar solution of an electrolyte has a higher osmotic pressure than a molar solution of a nonelectrolyte because the

      (A) electrolyte ions carry electric charges
      (B) electrolyte ions are usually hydrated
      (C) electrolyte alters the dielectric constant of water
      (D) electrolyte dissociates in solution
      (E) nonelectrolyte is not polar

8. The immediate precursor of urinary ammonia is

    (A) urea
    (B) uric acid
    (C) the amide nitrogen of glutamine
    (D) the epsilon-amino group of lysine
    (E) the alpha-amino nitrogen of glutamic acid

9. The fourth cranial or trochlear nerve innervates

    (A) the lacrimal gland
    (B) a muscle that turns the eyeball superiorly and laterally
    (C) the medial part of the lower eyelid
    (D) a muscle that turns the eyeball inferiorly and laterally
    (E) the lacrimal caruncle

10. A patient's left upper eyelid droops, his left eyeball is apparently recessed, and his left pupil is constricted. The left side of his face is flushed but dry. Which of the following is the most likely diagnosis?

    (A) A tumor in the interpeduncular fossa pressing forward on the posterior hypothalamic nuclei and backward on the left oculomotor nerve
    (B) A tumor in the pretectal region
    (C) A tumor pressing on the cervical sympathetic trunk
    (D) An infarct of the branch of the middle cerebral artery supplying the middle region of the precentral gyrus of the frontal lobe
    (E) None of the above

11. In basal fractures of the skull, if cerebrospinal fluid escapes from the nose, there is probably a fracture of the

    (A) nasal bone
    (B) temporal bone
    (C) ethmoid bone
    (D) parietal bone
    (E) frontal bone

12. If a patient has received no preanesthetic medication and breathes a gas mixture of 80 per cent nitrous oxide and 20 per cent oxygen, which of the following is most likely to occur?

    (A) Severe damage to the brain, consequent to anoxia
    (B) Analgesia
    (C) Deep surgical anesthesia
    (D) Respiratory arrest
    (E) No obvious effect

13. Spinal transection at about T6 may be followed by hypotension resulting primarily from

    (A) impairment of sympathetic vasoconstriction
    (B) impairment of myocardial contraction
    (C) lack of proprioceptive input from the lower limbs
    (D) a decrease in the volume of circulating whole blood
    (E) none of the above

14. Loss of scattered anterior horn cells by amyotrophic lateral sclerosis
results in which of the following changes in a skeletal muscle such as
the deltoid?

    (A) Atrophy of single muscle fibers
    (B) Atrophy of muscle fibers of individual motor units
    (C) Diffuse atrophy of muscle fibers
    (D) Swelling and hyalinization of muscle fibers
    (E) Regenerative buds and increased sarcolemmal nuclei

15. In progressive muscular dystrophy, the essential pathological changes
occur

    (A) in anterior horn cells of the spinal cord
    (B) in motor fibers of peripheral nerves
    (C) in motor end-plates (myoneural junctions)
    (D) within muscle fibers
    (E) in the ground substance of muscular interstitium

16. In both sexes

    (A) the bladder in adults is confined to the true pelvis (pelvis
        minor)
    (B) the major source of blood to the rectum is from the middle
        rectal (hemorrhoidal) arteries
    (C) the small intestine may be in contact with the bladder
        (through peritoneum)
    (D) the median sacral artery cannot be ligated without serious
        effects
    (E) efferent (motor) fibers from the sacral levels of the spinal
        cord pass directly to the muscle of the bladder

17. Collagenous scarring is not commonly observed in the brain, but it is
present in most instances of

    (A) multiple sclerosis
    (B) amyotrophic lateral sclerosis
    (C) brain abscess
    (D) senile atrophy
    (E) Parkinson's disease (paralysis agitans)

18. A nontoxigenic strain of *Corynebacterium diphtheriae* can be made toxigenic by

  (A) growth in a medium containing an optimal concentration of iron
  (B) mutation
  (C) recombination with an F$^+$ strain of *C. diphtheriae*
  (D) lysogenic conversion
  (E) repeated intraperitoneal passage in susceptible animals

19. Death in diphtheria is usually caused by

  (A) laryngeal paralysis
  (B) hyperthermia
  (C) convulsions with brain damage
  (D) respiratory failure
  (E) myocardial failure

20. Which of the following processes is most likely to predispose to the development of a tubal pregnancy?

  (A) Tuberculous endometritis
  (B) Vaginitis related to trichomoniasis
  (C) Lymphopathia venereum
  (D) Syphilis
  (E) Gonococcal salpingitis

21. The bacterium that most frequently causes meningitis with a predominance of lymphocytes in spinal fluid is

  (A) *Neisseria meningitidis*
  (B) *Haemophilus influenzae*
  (C) *Staphylococcus aureus*
  (D) *Mycobacterium tuberculosis*
  (E) *Diplococcus pneumoniae*

22. The most practicable available method for controlling the spread of St. Louis encephalitis virus is

  (A) eradication of wild waterfowl
  (B) eradication of houseflies
  (C) vaccination of poultry flocks
  (D) intensive mosquito control
  (E) burning over marshlands

9

23. The principal reason for administering live poliovirus vaccine on a 3-dose schedule is to

   (A) reduce the chance of interference among poliovirus types
   (B) provide a booster or anamnestic response
   (C) lessen neurotoxicity
   (D) permit continued clinical surveillance of the recipient
   (E) increase the opportunity for viral interference with wild-type enteroviruses

24. The effectiveness of interferon as an antiviral agent depends upon its ability to

   (A) combine with and neutralize extracellular virions
   (B) prevent the penetration of viruses into a cell
   (C) destroy the protein coat surrounding a virus
   (D) act intracellularly to prevent the production of new mature virions
   (E) stimulate the host defenses, leading to earlier and increased antibody production

25. The ineffectiveness of penicillins against fungi, protozoa, and viruses can be attributed to the

   (A) lack of sterols in membranes or envelopes
   (B) presence of sterols in membranes or envelopes
   (C) impermeability of cell membranes to penicillin
   (D) absence of mucopeptide-containing cell walls
   (E) production of penicillinase by these organisms

26. The basis for the toxic action of the polyene antibiotics (nystatin and amphotericin B) on microorganisms is dependent upon their binding to

   (A) sterols
   (B) lipoproteins
   (C) chitin
   (D) nucleic acids
   (E) polysaccharides

27. Complement is required in order to demonstrate

   (A) immune bacteriolysis
   (B) heterophil sheep-cell agglutination
   (C) the agar gel diffusion reaction
   (D) typhoid O agglutinins
   (E) diphtheria toxin-antitoxin flocculation

28. The mechanism by which antihistaminic compounds relieve allergic conditions involves

    (A) acceleration of the excretion of histamine
    (B) neutralization of the effects of histamine by producing the opposite reactions
    (C) chemical combination with histamine and inactivation of it
    (D) competition with histamine in attachment to cell receptors
    (E) activation of histamine oxidase

29. In intracartilaginous ossification, the osteoblasts initially deposit bone on

    (A) living cartilage cells
    (B) the collagenous matrix
    (C) dead cartilage cells
    (D) interstitial lamellae of bone
    (E) the calcified cartilage matrix

30. Administration of luteinizing hormone to a male causes

    (A) increased spermatogenesis
    (B) stimulation of androgen secretion by cells of the seminiferous tubules
    (C) secretion of androgen by interstitial cells of the testes
    (D) contraction of the epididymis
    (E) increased motility of Leydig's cells

DIRECTIONS: This section of the test consists of situations, each followed by a series of questions. Study each situation, and select the one best answer to each question following it.

Questions 31–34

A 68-year-old physician, apparently well except for mild diabetes mellitus and essential hypertension (blood pressure 160/95 mm Hg), both of about 10 years' duration, felt severe crushing precordial pain while shoveling snow. He collapsed and was taken to a hospital, where he was found to be in shock and cyanotic with hypotension and a rapid, feeble pulse. Given oxygen and supportive therapy, he improved somewhat, his blood pressure returning to its former level. Six days after admission, while using the bed pan, the patient died suddenly. At autopsy, extensive myocardial infarction was found.

31. Examination of the kidneys would be most likely to disclose

    (A) acute pyelonephritis
    (B) acute glomerulonephritis
    (C) benign nephrosclerosis
    (D) malignant nephrosclerosis
    (E) chronic glomerulonephritis

32. The most likely cause of the myocardial infarction was

    (A) syphilitic aortitis with occlusion of a coronary orifice
    (B) embolus to a coronary artery
    (C) dissecting aneurysm with occlusion of a coronary orifice
    (D) occlusion of a coronary orifice due to atheroma
    (E) coronary thrombus on the basis of an atheroma

33. Histologically, the prominent feature of the infarct might have been any of the following EXCEPT

    (A) necrotic muscle
    (B) infiltration by polymorphonuclear leukocytes
    (C) replacement of muscle by fibrous tissue
    (D) fibrinous exudate on the pericardium
    (E) unorganized endocardial thrombus

34. One might expect to find each of the following EXCEPT

    (A) fibrinous pericarditis
    (B) verrucous endocarditis
    (C) endocardial thrombus
    (D) rupture of the myocardium
    (E) cardiac dilatation

Questions 35–39

An overdose of a new drug produced progressive effects referable to the central nervous system including vertigo, ataxia, somnolence, hypnosis and respiratory depression. These began within 15 minutes after oral administration of the drug. No metabolic breakdown products were found in the urine; however, a high concentration of the agent was found in the bile.

The following information was obtained from the manufacturer: The drug is an organic acid with a pK$_a$ of 6.4 and high lipid solubility; the drug is excreted by humans in such a way that one half of the administered drug is eliminated in the urine within three days.

35. The symptoms and physicochemical data indicate that the drug probably

    (A) passes readily through cell membranes, including the blood-brain barrier
    (B) passes readily through cell membranes but does not pass the blood-brain barrier
    (C) penetrates readily from the circulation into the brain but not into other organs
    (D) can diffuse only into the glomerular filtrate
    (E) cannot escape from the circulation

36. The information that the drug is highly concentrated in bile suggests

    (A) that the drug is probably efficiently excreted in the feces
    (B) that the drug is probably structurally similar to a bile acid
    (C) that the drug forms complexes with bile acids
    (D) that the drug is effectively absorbed from the large intestine
    (E) none of the above conclusions

37. The fact that it takes three days for half of the drug to appear in the urine is best explained on the basis that the drug

    (A) is bound to plasma protein
    (B) undergoes little or no metabolism and is passively reabsorbed from the renal tubules
    (C) is deposited in bone
    (D) is actively secreted by the renal tubules
    (E) does none of the above

38. The ratio of the unionized to the ionized form of the drug in plasma at pH 7.4 is

    (A) 1:10
    (B) 1:1
    (C) 10:1
    (D) 100:1
    (E) 1000:1

39. Acidification of the urine by administration of ammonium sulfate would

    (A) increase the relative concentration of the ionized form of the drug in tubular fluid, which is likely to increase urinary excretion

    (B) increase the relative concentration of the ionized form of the drug, which is likely to decrease urinary excretion

    (C) decrease the relative concentration of the ionized form of the drug, which is likely to increase urinary excretion

    (D) decrease the relative concentration of the ionized form of the drug, which is likely to decrease urinary excretion

    (E) increase secretion of the drug by the renal tubules

Questions 40–42

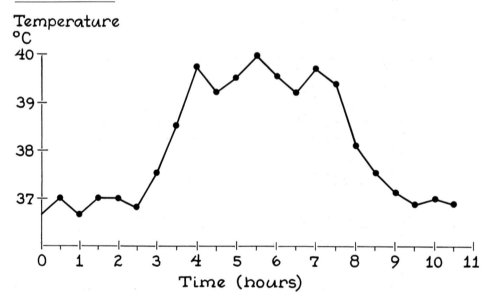

The figure above shows the time course of a typical febrile episode as recorded from a rectal thermometer.

40. During the onset of the febrile period,

    (A) the elevation in body temperature is promptly sensed by hypothalamic thermal receptors that activate cooling mechanisms

    (B) cutaneous warm receptors are relatively active

    (C) sweating and vasodilation appear promptly

    (D) the patient responds physiologically through mechanisms ordinarily activated by a cold environment

    (E) a breakdown in thermogenesis takes place

41. During the period of sustained fever,

      (A) regulatory adjustments are maintained but are less precise
      (B) heat production steadily exceeds heat loss
      (C) total heat loss steadily exceeds heat production
      (D) radiative and convective heat losses are markedly reduced
      (E) the hypothalamic "thermostat" is reset at an abnormally low value

42. In producing fever of this type, endogenous pyrogens in the blood

      (A) act upon skeletal muscle to increase metabolic activity
      (B) directly inhibit secretory activity of the sweat glands
      (C) directly induce both shivering and vasodilation
      (D) act to reset the hypothalamic "thermostat" to regulate at a higher temperature
      (E) directly attack and destroy infectious disease organisms

---

DIRECTIONS: Each group of questions below consists of five lettered headings or a diagram or table with five lettered components, followed by a list of numbered words, phrases or statements. For each numbered word, phrase or statement, select the one lettered heading or lettered component that is most closely associated with it. Each lettered heading or lettered component may be selected once, more than once, or not at all.

Questions 43–45

For each region, indicate the epithelium that would usually be expected.

      (A) Stratified squamous
      (B) Transitional
      (C) Simple columnar
      (D) Simple cuboidal
      (E) Pseudostratified ciliated columnar

43. The primary bronchus

44. The ileocolic junction

45. The proximal part of the female urethra

Questions 46–48

(A) Bacterial flagellum
(B) Mitochondrion
(C) Cell membrane
(D) Wall of a gram-positive bacterium
(E) Wall of a gram-negative bacterium

46. The location of cytochrome enzymes in bacteria

47. The location of teichoic acids

48. An entity composed exclusively of protein

Questions 49–51

(A) Amphotericin B
(B) Nystatin
(C) Neomycin
(D) Griseofulvin
(E) Bacitracin

49. An antifungal agent effective in the treatment of systemic mycoses

50. An antifungal agent effective in the treatment of ringworm of the skin and nails

51. An agent used primarily in the treatment of Candida infections of the skin, mucous membrane and intestinal tract

Questions 52–54

(A) Nitrogen mustard
(B) ^{32}P
(C) Methotrexate (Amethopterin)
(D) 6-Mercaptopurine
(E) Colchicine

52. A hypoxanthine analog

53. An agent which interrupts mitotic activity at the metaphase

54. An alkylating agent

Questions 55–58

Patient	Distressful Signs or Symptoms	Respiratory Minute Vol. (1/minute)	Urinary pH	Urinary 24-Hour vol. (ml)	Na+	Plasma (mEq/1)		
						K+	Cl-	HCO3-
Normal	None	8	6.8	2000	140	5	100	27
(A)	Shortness of breath	5	6.0	2100	141	5.1	94	34
(B)	Weakness	7.8	7.3	1800	129	7	92	26
(C)	Hyperpnea	10	5.8	4000	124	5.1	90	11
(D)	Dizziness and muscle twitching	16	7.6	2200	134	4.9	105	22
(E)	Thirst	8	7.2	15,000	165	5.5	125	27

The table above presents information concerning the respiratory, renal, and acid-base states of several different patients in relation to values approximating those found in normal men. For each question, select the letter designating the patient most likely to be represented by the situation described.

55. The patient has a plasma pH significantly greater than normal

56. The patient is experiencing interference with the free movement of air in respiratory passageways

57. The patient has been experiencing excessive metabolic production of acids, such as acetoacetic acid, possibly due to unregulated diabetes mellitus

58. The patient has an inadequately functioning posterior pituitary gland

Questions 59–62

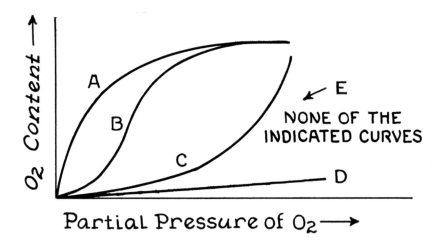

Each of the lettered curves shown above may depict a relationship of the total content of oxygen in solution to the partial pressure of oxygen.

59. Shape of the curve that represents the relationship of oxygen contained in physical solution in plasma to the partial pressure of oxygen

60. Shape of the curve that would be observed for the reversible binding of oxygen to normal human myoglobin

61. Shape of the curve that would be observed for the reversible binding of oxygen to normal human hemoglobin

62. Shape of the curve that would be observed for the binding of oxygen to an abnormal human hemoglobin that lacks heme-heme interaction

Questions 63–67

DIRECTION OF ARROW indicates change from average normal values; 0 indicates absence of change from normal.

	ARTERIAL BLOOD		MIXED VENOUS BLOOD	
	O_2 content ml/100 ml	P_{O_2} mm Hg	O_2 content ml/100 ml	P_{O_2} mm Hg
(A)	↓	↓	↓	↓
(B)	0	0	↑	↑
(C)	↓	↑	↓	↓
(D)	↑	↑	↓	↓
(E)	↓	0	↓	↓

63. Iron-deficiency anemia

64. A femoral arteriovenous fistula

65. Acute respiratory failure in poliomyelitis

66. Nonfatal carbon-monoxide poisoning

67. Severe barbiturate poisoning

Questions 68–71

A study of intermediary metabolism has revealed that most vitamins function as the precursors of coenzymes or prosthetic groups. For each numbered item, select the vitamin involved in its formation.

(A) Thiamine
(B) Nicotinamide
(C) Vitamin C
(D) Vitamin B$_6$
(E) Pantothenic acid

68. Diphosphopyridine nucleotide

69. Pyridoxal phosphate

70. Cocarboxylase

71. Coenzyme A

DIRECTIONS: Each set of lettered headings below is followed by a list of numbered words or phrases. For each numbered word or phrase select

A   if the item is associated with (A) only,
B   if the item is associated with (B) only,
C   if the item is associated with both (A) and (B),
D   if the item is associated with neither (A) nor (B).

Questions 72–75

    (A) Cellular proliferation continually renews the cellular population in adults

    (B) Cellular proliferation occurs or increases sporadically to compensate for injury or to meet increased functional demands

    (C) Both

    (D) Neither

72. Neurons

73. Intestinal absorptive cells

74. Hepatic parenchymal cells

75. Epidermis

Questions 76–78

    (A) Chronic granulocytic leukemia

    (B) Acute leukemia

    (C) Both

    (D) Neither

76. Chromosomal errors in leukemic cells

77. Ph^1 (Philadelphia) chromosome (G group deletion)

78. Down's syndrome (mongolism)

DIRECTIONS: For each of the questions or incomplete statements below, ONE or MORE of the answers or completions given is correct. Select

    A if only 1, 2, and 3 are correct,

    B if only 1 and 3 are correct,

    C if only 2 and 4 are correct,

    D if only 4 is correct,

    E if all are correct.

Directions Summarized				
A	B	C	D	E
1,2,3 only	1,3 only	2,4 only	4 only	All are correct

79. The molecular weight of a protein may be estimated by

    (1) infrared analysis
    (2) ultracentrifugation
    (3) electrophoresis
    (4) gel filtration

80. Forces or bonds that may be important in determining the three-dimensional structure of proteins include

    (1) covalent bonds
    (2) electrostatic attraction and repulsion forces
    (3) hydrogen bonds
    (4) hydrophobic bonds

81. The immunogenicity of macromolecules generally

    (1) is greatest for proteins
    (2) involves the recognition of the macromolecule as foreign to the host
    (3) depends on the route of administration
    (4) is enhanced by prior enzymatic fragmentation

82. Subcutaneous injections of one's own tissues from which of the following would induce the production of autoantibodies?

    (1) Brain
    (2) Thyroid
    (3) Spermatozoa
    (4) Uterine muscle

83. A reaction of the delayed type occurs in the

    (1) tuberculin skin test
    (2) Schick test
    (3) mumps skin test
    (4) ragweed pollen skin test

84. The classical Arthus' reaction is associated with

    (1) the presence of precipitating antibodies
    (2) migration of polymorphonuclear leukocytes to the reaction site
    (3) fixation of complement to the antigen-antibody aggregate
    (4) histamine release

Directions Summarized				
A	B	C	D	E
1,2,3 only	1,3 only	2,4 only	4 only	All are correct

85. Genetic resistance of bacteria to antibiotics can be acquired by

    (1) the uptake of DNA extracted from resistant cells of the same species
    (2) phage-mediated transduction from resistant donors
    (3) the conjugational transfer of an episome
    (4) mutation specifically induced by the antibiotic

86. Cholera is characterized by

    (1) liquid stools low in protein and high in potassium and bicarbonate
    (2) hemoconcentration, acidosis, and hypokalemia
    (3) paralysis of the sodium-potassium pump of the intestinal mucosa
    (4) blood cultures positive for *Vibrio cholerae*

87. Capsules of the pneumococci

    (1) consist of lipopolysaccharide, protein, and carbohydrate
    (2) stimulate the formation of protective antibodies
    (3) are most likely to be found on pneumococci grown in the presence of type-specific antipneumococcal antibody
    (4) are required for virulence

88. Reactions in which there is a net loss of an energy-rich phosphate bond include

    (1) 1,3-diphosphoglyceric acid $+ H O \rightarrow$ 3-phosphoglyceric acid $+$ inorganic phosphate
    (2) $ATP + creatine \rightarrow creatine\text{-}phosphate + ADP$
    (3) $ATP + glucose \rightarrow glucose\text{-}6\text{-}phosphate + ADP$
    (4) $2\text{-}ADP \rightarrow ATP + AMP$

Directions Summarized				
A	B	C	D	E
1,2,3 only	1,3 only	2,4 only	4 only	All are correct

89. In Type I glycogen storage disease (glucose-6-phosphate deficiency), there is an abnormally large accumulation of glycogen in the

    (1) liver
    (2) cardiac muscle
    (3) kidneys
    (4) skeletal muscle

90. Enzymes

    (1) increase the rate of a reaction
    (2) lower the activation energy of a reaction
    (3) act specifically on one substrate or a group of related substrates
    (4) alter the equilibrium constant of a reaction

91. The pK_a of lactic acid is 3.85. A buffer could be prepared at this pH by the addition of

    (1) 50 ml of 0.1 N sodium hydroxide to 100 ml of 0.1 N lactic acid
    (2) 100 ml 0.1 N sodium lactate to 50 ml of 0.2 N lactic acid
    (3) 50 ml of 0.2 N sodium lactate to 50 ml of 0.1 N hydrochloric acid
    (4) 50 ml of 0.2 N sodium hydroxide to 50 ml of 0.1 N lactic acid

92. The major mechanisms for the termination of norepinephrine action in the body include

    (1) methylation to 3-methoxy-norepinephrine (normetanephrine) by the enzyme catechol-O-methyl transferase (COMT)
    (2) deamination to 3,4-dihydroxymandelic acid by the enzyme monoamine oxidase (MAO)
    (3) uptake by nerve endings
    (4) N-methylation to epinephrine

Directions Summarized				
A	B	C	D	E
1,2,3 only	1,3 only	2,4 only	4 only	All are correct

93. Extracts of the hypothalamus act on the pituitary gland to

    (1) increase the output of ACTH

    (2) increase the uptake of ^{131}I by the thyroid gland by increasing the output of thyroid-stimulating hormone

    (3) stimulate ovulation from mature follicles by increasing the output of luteinizing hormone

    (4) decrease the output of prolactin

94. Drugs used to treat acute leukemia include

    (1) 6-mercaptopurine

    (2) aminopterin

    (3) cortisone

    (4) folic acid

95. Accumulation of fat in hepatic parenchymal cells can be induced by

    (1) a dietary deficiency of lipotropic factors

    (2) protein deficiency

    (3) ingestion of halogenated hydrocarbons

    (4) chronic ingestion of alcohol

96. Mesoderm in the early embryo is the germ layer source of

    (1) macrophages

    (2) lung epithelium

    (3) pericardium

    (4) hair follicles

97. In the mammalian kidney, urea

    (1) is freely filtrable at the glomerulus

    (2) is actively transported into the proximal tubule

    (3) has a clearance less than that of inulin

    (4) is excreted at a rate independent of the rate of urine flow

Directions Summarized				
A	B	C	D	E
1,2,3 only	1,3 only	2,4 only	4 only	All are correct

98. The venous return to the heart increases transiently when

    (1) a sudden increase in blood volume occurs
    (2) the abdomen is suddenly compressed
    (3) the sympathetics are suddenly stimulated
    (4) the arterioles suddenly constrict

99. Which of the following vessels usually anastomose with one another and together form a chief supply to the parts named?

    (1) The right gastric and the left gastric arteries supplying the lesser curvature of the stomach
    (2) The superior pancreaticoduodenal and the inferior pancreaticoduodenal arteries supplying the tail of the pancreas
    (3) The right colic artery and the ileocolic artery supplying the appendix
    (4) The left colic artery and the middle colic artery supplying the right (hepatic) flexure of the large intestine

100. Toxic doses of digitoxin may produce

    (1) anorexia
    (2) disturbances of color vision
    (3) ventricular extrasystoles
    (4) vomiting

Part II—Examples of Questions Drawn From
Clinical Subjects: Questions 1–100

DIRECTIONS: Each of the questions or incomplete statements below is followed by five suggested answers or completions. Select the one that is BEST in each case.

1. The life expectancy for white females born in 1960 was 73 years. This means that

  (A) the average age at death among white females in 1960 was 73 years
  (B) the life span of white females in 1960 was 73 years
  (C) under mortality conditions in 1960, every white female may expect to live at least 73 years
  (D) the average life expectancy of white females at all ages in 1960 was 73 years
  (E) on the average, white females would live 73 years if the age-specific death rates for white females in 1960 continue unchanged throughout their lives

2. Life expectancy has increased markedly in the United States during the past 50 years chiefly because of

  (A) a continued reduction in the death rates of infants and children
  (B) the continuous decline in tuberculosis
  (C) the fact that older adults reach retirement age in better health
  (D) a fairly uniform reduction of death rates in all age groups
  (E) control of industrial health hazards

3. In acute intestinal obstruction due to incarcerated hernia, the spasms of pain result from

  (A) constriction of the bowel at the site of obstruction
  (B) necrosis of the bowel at the site of obstruction
  (C) inflammatory exudate soiling the peritoneal surfaces
  (D) contraction of the distended bowel above the site of obstruction
  (E) compression of the nerves of the bowel

4. A patient with a history of fever and mild diarrhea of two months' duration is found to have a palpable mass in the right lower quadrant of the abdomen. The most likely diagnosis is

    (A) regional enteritis
    (B) ulcerative colitis
    (C) amebic colitis
    (D) diverticulitis
    (E) lymphoma

5. Uterine retroversion is

    (A) often a cause of pelvic pain
    (B) relatively infrequent
    (C) usually associated with a lumbar backache
    (D) usually asymptomatic
    (E) a cause of endometriosis

6. The decline in the reported deaths from cancer of the stomach is most likely to be the result of

    (A) improved methods of treatment
    (B) changes in death certificate classification
    (C) earlier diagnosis
    (D) lower incidence
    (E) none of the above

7. A 22-year-old multipara, who has had a successful removal of a small intraepithelial carcinoma of the cervix by wide conization, would like to have more children. Management should consist of

    (A) regular pelvic examinations and Papanicolaou smears
    (B) small amounts of radium therapy to the cervix with the ovaries shielded
    (C) annual curettage
    (D) cervical amputation
    (E) administration of progesterone

8. Which of the following, if persistent, is usually incompatible with spontaneous delivery at term?

    (A) Mentum posterior
    (B) Mentum anterior
    (C) Sacrum posterior
    (D) Occiput posterior
    (E) Caput succedaneum

9. Of the following, primary amenorrhea is most commonly caused by

    (A) pregnancy
    (B) ovarian tumors
    (C) congenital abnormalities
    (D) tuberculosis
    (E) lactation

10. The excretion of pregnanediol glucuronide usually

    (A) reaches maximum values during menstruation
    (B) decreases immediately before menstruation
    (C) is uninfluenced by follicle development
    (D) is not related to the menstrual cycle
    (E) varies inversely with progesterone secretion

11. During the climacteric, the urinary excretion of gonadotropin tends to

    (A) increase
    (B) decrease
    (C) vary directly with ovarian function
    (D) remain unaltered
    (E) show unpredictable and great variations

12. In the prevention of cardiovalvular disease in a child who has had rheumatic fever, the most important principle is

    (A) insistence on complete bed rest until the erythrocyte sedimentation rate has returned to normal
    (B) prevention of subsequent attacks of rheumatic fever by drug prophylaxis
    (C) adequate treatment with corticosteroids during acute attacks of rheumatic fever
    (D) adequate prophylactic and restorative dental care to forestall the formation of periodontal abscess or infection
    (E) none of the above

13. A large peripheral arteriovenous fistula should produce a decreased

    (A) pulse rate
    (B) cardiac output
    (C) diastolic blood pressure
    (D) heart size
    (E) venous pressure distal to the fistula

14. A left varicocele which develops after a patient is more than 30 years old and does not collapse when the patient lies supine is indicative of obstruction of the

    (A) pampiniform plexus
    (B) splenic vein
    (C) left renal vein
    (D) vena cava below the renal veins
    (E) left internal iliac vein

15. An appropriate surgical operation is most likely to provide effective relief of ascites when the ascites is secondary to

    (A) cirrhosis of the liver with esophageal varices
    (B) constrictive pericarditis
    (C) tricuspid insufficiency
    (D) thrombosis of the portal vein
    (E) hepatic vein thrombosis (Budd-Chiari syndrome)

16. Following resuscitation from cardiac arrest, a patient is found to have

Arterial pH	7.00
Arterial $P_O{}^2$	40 mm Hg
Arterial P_{CO}	50 mm Hg
Plasma HCO_3	8.0 mEq/l
Serum Na^+	145 mEq/l
Serum K^+	6.0 mEq/l

Which of the following statements concerning this patient is most accurate?

    (A) The plasma Cl^- is greater than 110 mEq/l
    (B) The degree of acidosis is determined by the patient's hypercapnia
    (C) The increased plasma K^+ reflects acute renal failure
    (D) The plasma Cl^- is less than 85 mEq/l
    (E) The plasma lactate is greater than 10 mEq/l

17. Hereditary nephropathy may be strongly suspected in the face of recurrent hematuria, a family history of renal disease, and

    (A) deafness
    (B) renal rickets
    (C) azotemia
    (D) bicuspid aortic valve
    (E) horseshoe kidney

18. A 64-year-old diabetic woman enters the hospital with a high fever, back pain, and hematuria. Six months prior to her acute illness her blood urea nitrogen was noted to be 25 mg/100 ml. On admission her BUN is 100 mg/100 ml. Examination of the urine shows numerous gram-negative rods, 1+ protein, 10-25 erythrocytes per high-power field, and numerous hyaline and granular casts. Despite treatment with fluids and antibiotic agents, her fever continues and she develops progressive azotemia. The probable diagnosis is

   (A) acute tubular necrosis
   (B) Kimmelstiel-Wilson syndrome
   (C) renal venous thrombosis
   (D) necrotizing papillitis
   (E) renal cortical necrosis

19. A 65-year-old man, previously well adjusted, began to show a tendency to isolate himself and to be suspicious of others after he had developed tinnitus and progressive loss of hearing. The history suggests

   (A) an early schizophrenic reaction
   (B) organic brain syndrome
   (C) cerebral arteriosclerosis
   (D) psychological reaction to deafness
   (E) none of the above

20. A 36-year-old obese man becomes progressively more elated and excited with increasing capacity for work. He becomes humorous and overactive to the point where it irritates others. He is probably suffering from

   (A) catatonic excitement
   (B) hypomania
   (C) panic reaction
   (D) alcoholic intoxication
   (E) agitated depression

21. Paranoid delusions involve which of the following psychological defense mechanisms?

   (A) Conversion and displacement
   (B) Denial and projection
   (C) Identification with the aggressor
   (D) Isolation and regression
   (E) Repression

22. Which of the following suggests an unfavorable prognosis in schizo-phrenia?

    (A) No obvious precipitating factors
    (B) Abrupt onset
    (C) Intense affect
    (D) Changing symptoms
    (E) Short duration of symptoms

23. If the sensitivity of a screening test for a defined disease is 95 per cent, it may be expected that

    (A) the test will be positive in 95 per cent of individuals with the disease
    (B) the test will be negative in 95 per cent of individuals without the disease
    (C) of the positive individuals, 95 per cent will have the disease
    (D) of the negative individuals, no more than 5 per cent will have the disease
    (E) none of the above is true

24. If the case-fatality rate in a test group receiving a new drug is lower than that in a control group by an amount that is statistically significant at the 5 per cent level, it follows that the

    (A) better results in the test group are attributed to the new drug
    (B) chances are less than one in twenty that the difference is due to sampling variation
    (C) difference could not be due to chance
    (D) chances are more than twenty to one that the difference is due to sampling variation
    (E) drug had no effect on mortality

25. By the application of appropriate statistical techniques to data collected in the course of an experiment, one can usually

    (A) eliminate the influence of chance factors upon the results of the experiment
    (B) estimate the probability that the results obtained could have occurred by chance alone
    (C) reduce the amount of variability present in the data
    (D) control for the effects of sampling errors upon the results of the experiment
    (E) determine whether or not cause-and-effect relationships exist among the variables being studied

26. In an investigation of data on the use of an immunizing agent, the application of a statistical test of significance indicates

   (A) whether the sample size was large enough to provide meaningful results
   (B) the extent to which the agent was probably effective in producing any observed differences
   (C) that bias was eliminated
   (D) how often results would differ by as much as the observed difference if chance alone were operating
   (E) the probability that the agent was effective

27. In a child suspected of having acute disseminated histoplasmosis, which of the following tests would be likely to yield the most helpful information?

   (A) Sheep-cell agglutination titer
   (B) Examination of the bone marrow aspirate
   (C) Skull roentgenogram
   (D) Sedimentation rate
   (E) Widal reaction

28. A 35-year-old farmer sustained a deep puncture wound in his left thigh when he fell on the prongs of a manure fork. You attend him within two hours of the injury, which has produced no serious vascular or neurological problems. After debridement of the wound you should immediately administer

   (A) a broad-spectrum antibiotic agent (with the expectation of continuing it)
   (B) 10,000 units of equine tetanus antitoxin
   (C) 16,000 units of equine tetanus antitoxin
   (D) 1 ml of tetanus toxoid and 500 units of human antitetanus globulin
   (E) 2 ml of *Clostridium perfringens* toxoid

29. Which of the following is LEAST likely to accompany posterior dislocation of the hip?

   (A) Aseptic necrosis of the head of the femur
   (B) A chip fracture of the ipsilateral acetabular lip
   (C) Hemarthrosis of the ipsilateral knee
   (D) Damage to the sciatic nerve
   (E) Damage to the femoral nerve

30. Once carcinoma of the lung has been diagnosed, each of the following is usually considered a sign of inoperability EXCEPT

   (A) paralysis of the diaphragm on the ipsilateral side
   (B) Horner's syndrome on the ipsilateral side
   (C) serosanguineous pleural effusion
   (D) marked pulmonary osteoarthropathy
   (E) biopsy of an anterior scalene node that is positive for tumor

31. The probability of postpartum hemorrhage is increased by each of the following EXCEPT

   (A) precipitate labor
   (B) prolonged labor
   (C) multiple pregnancy
   (D) premature rupture of the membranes
   (E) hydramnios

32. Congestive heart failure is associated with each of the following EXCEPT

   (A) decreased renal blood flow
   (B) increased blood volume
   (C) hypernatremia
   (D) increased interstitial fluid volume
   (E) decreased glomerular filtration rate

33. A 48-year-old patient with a history suggestive of an indolent, progressive meningitis of two weeks' duration shows signs of meningeal irritation. Lumbar puncture yields slightly cloudy fluid with 380 leukocytes (90 per cent lymphocytes, 10 per cent polymorphonuclear cells); protein 110 mg/100 ml; glucose 10 mg/100 ml. Each of the following etiologic possibilities might be seriously considered in the differential diagnosis EXCEPT

   (A) *Cryptococcus neoformans*
   (B) *Mycobacterium tuberculosis*
   (C) lymphomatous involvement of the meninges
   (D) Coxsackie virus, group B
   (E) carcinomatous involvement of the meninges

34. Each of the following may promote convulsive seizures in susceptible individuals EXCEPT

    (A) acidosis
    (B) hypoglycemia
    (C) excessive water retention
    (D) alkalosis
    (E) withdrawal of phenobarbital

35. Each of the following is associated with intrauterine growth retardation of the fetus EXCEPT

    (A) trisomy 17-18
    (B) rubella
    (C) osteogenesis imperfecta
    (D) cystic fibrosis
    (E) toxoplasmosis

DIRECTIONS: This section of the test consists of several situations, each followed by a series of questions. Study each situation, and select the one best answer to each question following it.

Questions 36–37

A physician is called to an apartment to see a new patient. He finds the markedly jaundiced body of a young woman, whose alleged sister gives the following history. Five days previously the patient, who thought she was pregnant, had gone to see a man who inserted a catheter into the uterus to produce an abortion. Following this, she became very ill. She died shortly after the sister called the physician.

36. The physician should immediately

    (A) call in a consulting obstetrician
    (B) send the body to the nearest hospital for an autopsy
    (C) sign the death certificate, giving the cause of death as "abortion"
    (D) notify the police and await their instructions
    (E) send the body to the nearest mortuary and call the police

37. The most likely underlying cause of death is

     (A) liver failure
     (B) *Clostridium perfringens* septicemia
     (C) acute glomerulonephritis
     (D) *Escherichia coli* septicemia
     (E) *Staphylococcus aureus* septicemia

Questions 38–40

A 28-year-old drug addict is found in his room disoriented and covered with urine and feces. He is withdrawn and refuses to give a history. Physical examination shows a temperature of 40.9 C (105.6 F), a pulse rate of 132/min, a respiration rate of 24/min, and a blood pressure of 120/60 mm Hg. Surface veins of the forearms and upper arms are thrombosed and there are needle marks in both antecubital fossae. The heart, lungs, and abdomen show no abnormalities. He is admitted to the hospital with a presumptive diagnosis of bacterial endocarditis.

38. On the second hospital day, blood cultures taken on admission are reported as positive. The organism most likely to have been grown is

     (A) hemolytic (coagulase-positive) staphylococcus
     (B) *Staphylococcus epidermidis*
     (C) *Candida albicans*
     (D) group A beta-hemolytic streptococcus
     (E) streptococcus, viridans group

39. On the fourth hospital day, a harsh systolic murmur is heard over the center of the precordium, an enlarged pulsatile liver is felt, the neck veins are distended, and an infiltration of the right lower lobe is seen on a roentgenogram of the chest. The most likely explanation is

     (A) pulmonary hypertension secondary to multiple septic pulmonary emboli
     (B) rupture of an aneurysm of the sinus of Valsalva
     (C) purulent pericarditis
     (D) tricuspid valvular incompetence
     (E) mitral valvular incompetence

40. The best way to ascertain the nature of the anatomic lesion is by

(A) fluoroscopy
(B) right-heart catheterization with angiography
(C) right-heart catheterization with determination of pressures
    and flows
(D) left-heart catheterization with determination of pressures
    and flows
(E) left-heart catheterization with angiography

Questions 41–42

A 32-year-old man was getting gasoline at a roadside service station when
a car traveling at a high rate of speed hurtled from the road and crashed
into the automobile which the patient had vacated moments earlier. The
wreck burst into flame and, anticipating a serious explosion, the patient
assisted in pulling the driver from the flaming wreckage. An elderly man
who was helping the patient suffered a heart attack and died in the process,
and the extricated driver died moments later.

After the patient left the scene of the disaster, he was unable to stop
trembling, and he maintained a marked, visible tremor for two months,
during which time he had repetitive dreams of fighting his way out of a
raging fire which occurred in various settings.

41. The most likely diagnosis is

(A) hypochondriasis
(B) anxiety hysteria
(C) traumatic neurosis
(D) phobic reaction
(E) psychophysiological muscle reaction

42. The patient's repetitive dreams of fighting his way out of a fire prob-
     ably represent

(A) an attempt to master his anxiety
(B) his feeling of pleasure in being a hero
(C) a recollection of childhood incidents of playing with fire
(D) a wish to punish himself
(E) psychotic perseveration

Questions 43–45

A newborn infant with an abnormality of the genitalia that appears to be hypospadias is well for a week. Then the infant begins to vomit forcefully and becomes dehydrated. Administration of fluid and electrolytes parenterally in quantities usually sufficient to correct dehydration in a child of this age for at least a day fails to do so. Six hours after administration of the fluids the dehydration recurs, although the vomiting has stopped. A diagnosis of adrenal insufficiency associated with congenital adrenal hyperplasia is made.

43. At the time the dehydration was the greatest, the serum would be most likely to show

    (A) decreased carbon dioxide combining power and hyperchloremia

    (B) increased carbon dioxide combining power and hypochloremia

    (C) decreased carbon dioxide combining power and hypokalemia

    (D) hypochloremia, hyponatremia, hyperkalemia, and azotemia

    (E) no significant change from normal values

44. From the standpoint of diagnosis, the most important abnormality in the urine would be

    (A) marked reduction in specific gravity

    (B) absence or marked decrease of ammonia

    (C) increased excretion of 17-ketosteroids

    (D) marked decrease of chloride

    (E) a strongly acid reaction

45. In addition to parenteral administration of fluids and electrolytes, the preferred treatment would include

    (A) norepinephrine

    (B) vasopressin (Pitressin)

    (C) oral administration of a strongly alkaline electrolyte solution

    (D) ACTH

    (E) desoxycorticosterone acetate, supplemental salt, and cortisone

DIRECTIONS: Each group of questions below consists of lettered headings or a diagram or picture with lettered components, followed by a list of numbered words, phrases or statements. For each numbered word, phrase or statement, select the one lettered heading or lettered component most closely associated with it. Each lettered heading or lettered component may be selected once, more than once, or not at all.

Questions 46–49

The graphs below represent the patterns of labor in four different multiparous patients. For each statement that follows, select the pattern of labor most consistent with it, and mark the answer sheet in accordance with the following:

(A) if associated with graph A
(B) if associated with graph B
(C) if associated with graph C
(D) if associated with graph D

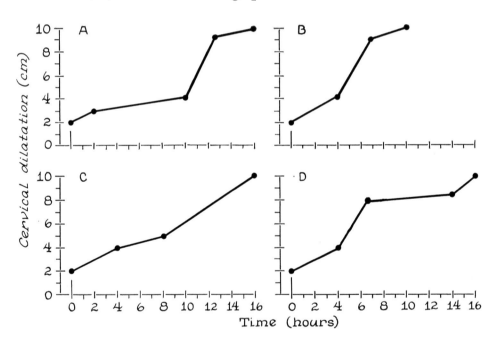

46. Secondary arrest

47. Normal labor

48. Prolonged latent phase

49. Desultory labor

Questions 50–54

Maternal history:

    (A) Oligohydramnios
    (B) Hydramnios
    (C) Toxemia
    (D) Diabetes mellitus
    (E) None of the above

Possible related condition in newborn:

50. Renal agenesis

51. Prematurity

52. Retrolental fibroplasia

53. Macrosomia

54. Duodenal atresia

Questions 55–59

    (A) Aseptic meningitis with a rash
    (B) Herpangina
    (C) Pharyngoconjunctival fever
    (D) Chorioretinitis
    (E) Epidemic pleurodynia

55. Coxsackie virus, group B

56. Toxoplasma

57. Adenovirus

58. ECHO virus

59. Coxsackie virus, group A

Questions 60–62

    (A) Vertical transmission
    (B) Indirect (vector) transmission
    (C) Transmission by a common vehicle through continuous exposure
    (D) Transmission by a common vehicle through a single exposure
    (E) Person-to-person transmission

60. Explosive outbreak

61. Secondary cases

62. Seasonal variation over a limited geographic area

Questions 63–66

    (A) Kanamycin sulfate
    (B) Tetracycline
    (C) Erythromycin
    (D) Chloroquine
    (E) Chloramphenicol

63. May cause hearing loss

64. Outdated material may cause aminoaciduria and renal tubular acidosis

65. May cause hemolytic anemia in genetically susceptible individuals

66. Prolonged therapy may cause proteinuria

Questions 67–70

Listed below are five lettered organs. For each of the numbered diseases that follow, select from the lettered list the organ other than the kidney that is most likely to be involved.

    (A) Lungs
    (B) Acoustic apparatus
    (C) Liver
    (D) Heart
    (E) Esophagus

67. Hereditary nephritis

68. Goodpasture's syndrome

69. Polycystic disease

70. Scleroderma

Questions 71–74

A patient is admitted to the emergency room following blunt trauma to the anterior chest wall. There are multiple fractured ribs on both sides of the sternum. Each of the lettered signs below is an additional finding that may be exhibited by this patient. For each of the numbered diagnoses that follow, select the sign that is most closely associated with it.

(A) Distended neck veins
(B) A "sucking" wound
(C) Paradoxical respiratory motion of the chest wall
(D) Subcutaneous emphysema
(E) A difference in blood pressure in the two arms

71. Flail chest

72. Cardiac tamponade

73. Tension pneumothorax

74. Lacerated lung

DIRECTIONS: Each set of lettered headings below is followed by a list of numbered words or phrases. For each numbered word or phrase select

A   if the item is associated with (A) only,
B   if the item is associated with (B) only,
C   if the item is associated with both (A) and (B),
D   if the item is associated with neither (A) nor (B).

Questions 75–76

(A) Patent ductus arteriosus
(B) Coarctation of the descending thoracic aorta
(C) Both
(D) Neither

75. Widened pulse pressure in the lower extremities

76. Can lead to left ventricular enlargement

11

Questions 77–81

      (A) Acute post-streptococcal glomerulonephritis
      (B) Acute rheumatic fever
      (C) Both
      (D) Neither

77. Reactivation frequently occurs in association with acquired streptococcal infection

78. Prolonged prophylactic administration of penicillin is recommended

79. Complete recovery without residual organ damage occurs in over 90 per cent of patients under 16 years of age

80. Infections with type 12 beta-hemolytic streptococci are particularly related

81. Electrocardiographic changes are seen

Questions 82–85

      (A) Rheumatic fever
      (B) Rheumatoid arthritis
      (C) Both
      (D) Neither

82. Antistreptolysin O titer elevated

83. Aortic regurgitation

84. Subcutaneous nodules

85. Therapy with penicillin relieves acute attack

DIRECTIONS: For each of the questions or incomplete statements below, ONE or MORE of the answers or completions given is correct. Select

A   if only 1, 2, and 3 are correct,

B   if only 1 and 3 are correct,

C   if only 2 and 4 are correct,

D   if only 4 is correct,

E   if all are correct.

		Directions Summarized		
A	B	C	D	E
1,2,3 only	1,3 only	2,4 only	4 only	All are correct

86. Which of the following may be useful in establishing the diagnosis of hypertension due to unilateral disease of a renal artery?

    (1) Aortography
    (2) Measurement of sodium excretion from each kidney
    (3) Intravenous pyelography
    (4) Measurement of plasma renin activity in blood from each renal vein

87. Intravenous pyelography is dangerous in a patient with

    (1) acute pyelonephritis
    (2) bilateral stag-horn calculi
    (3) an increased blood urea nitrogen concentration
    (4) allergy to iodides

88. Traumatic arteriovenous fistula produces

    (1) a wide pulse pressure
    (2) increased cardiac output
    (3) dilatation and hypertrophy of the left ventricle
    (4) pulmonary hypertension

89. An infant receiving a properly constructed formula of boiled cow's milk, water, and carbohydrate as his sole dietary intake would be prone to develop

    (1) kwashiorkor
    (2) anemia
    (3) beriberi
    (4) scurvy

90. Situations that tend to enhance the development of a strong ego during childhood include

    (1) exposure to frustrations that are rational and real rather than artificially created
    (2) exposure to frustrations that are, at the time, within the ego capacity of the child
    (3) repeated experiences with desirable substitute gratifications for forbidden and undesirable ones
    (4) minimizing, through explanation and affection, the tendency of the child to interpret reality frustrations as hostile attacks

91. A statistically significant association exists between perinatal traumata and

    (1) behavior disorders of childhood
    (2) hysterical reaction
    (3) epilepsy
    (4) somnambulism

92. In men with severe depressions, symptoms frequently include

    (1) early morning awakening
    (2) nihilistic delusions
    (3) diurnal mood swings
    (4) impotence

93. Compared with a suburban population, the population residing in the center of a large urban area has a significantly higher prevalence of

    (1) depression
    (2) schizophrenia
    (3) anxiety-hysteria
    (4) alcoholism

Directions Summarized				
A	B	C	D	E
1,2,3 only	1,3 only	2,4 only	4 only	All are correct

94. Choriocarcinoma

   (1) in many cases is successfully treated with methotrexate
   (2) will be a sequela of approximately 50 per cent of hydatidiform moles
   (3) can arise following an apparently normal pregnancy
   (4) produces excessive levels of follicle-stimulating hormone (FSH)

95. Palliation in metastatic carcinoma of the breast in a premenopausal woman may be achieved by

   (1) oophorectomy
   (2) hypophysectomy
   (3) adrenalectomy
   (4) administration of 5-fluorouracil

96. Compression of the first sacral root by a herniated lumbosacral disc produces

   (1) numbness of 5th toe
   (2) absence of the knee jerk
   (3) absence of the Achilles reflex
   (4) urinary retention

97. Oxytocin in humans is

   (1) a normally produced hormone with a polypeptide structure
   (2) rapidly eliminated or made inactive in both pregnant and nonpregnant patients
   (3) most effective at term in augmenting uterine contractions
   (4) released into the circulation as a result of suckling

Directions Summarized				
A	B	C	D	E
1,2,3 only	1,3 only	2,4 only	4 only	All are correct

98. A 13-year-old girl has had irregular, painless periods of uterine bleeding lasting as long as 12 days since the menarche nine months ago. Physical examination, including pelvic examination, shows no abnormalities. In this patient's premenstrual phase

   (1) premenstrual tension is unlikely
   (2) the endometrium is secretory
   (3) the cervical mucus shows a fern pattern
   (4) exfoliated vaginal cells curl and clump

99. Which of the following should not be used or should be used with caution in a patient suspected of having a duodenal ulcer?

   (1) Reserpine
   (2) Phenylbutazone
   (3) Cortisol
   (4) Aspirin

100. Normal immunologic responsiveness is depressed in patients with

   (1) a burn covering 40 per cent of the body surface
   (2) Hodgkin's disease
   (3) chronic uremia
   (4) myasthenia gravis, following thymectomy

Part III—Examples of Questions Presenting Clinical
Problems Based on Pictorial Material: Questions 1–18

DIRECTIONS: The questions below are related to accompanying illustrative material. Answer each question by selecting the one best choice.

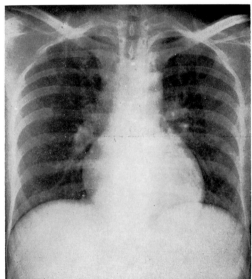
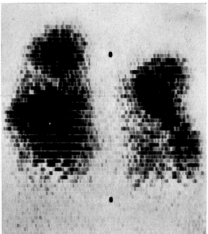

1. The above scan shows

    (A) areas of diminished alveolar ventilation
    (B) areas of diminished pulmonary perfusion
    (C) pulmonary consolidation
    (D) alveolar capillary block
    (E) localized area of overdistention

2. Which of the following is the most likely diagnosis?

    (A) Bullous emphysema
    (B) Pulmonary embolism
    (C) Pulmonary fibrosis
    (D) Pneumonia
    (E) Neoplastic disease

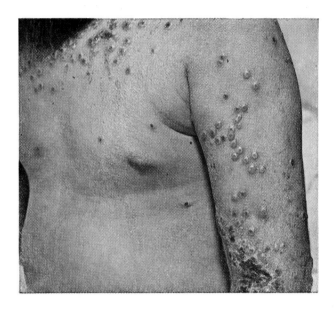

The above photograph is that of a 3-year-old boy who has had eczema for one year. Four days ago he developed vesiculopustular lesions in those areas of the face, neck, and arms where the eczema was most intense. He developed fever and, despite adequate penicillin therapy, new lesions continued to appear. Smears showed questionable intra-cytoplasmic inclusions but no multinucleated giant cells or intranuclear inclusions.

3. Which of the following statements would be most likely to apply?

    (A) The patient would improve dramatically when treated with erythromycin by mouth

    (B) A sister was vaccinated three weeks previously

    (C) Spherical particles would be found in vesicle fluid by electron microscopy

    (D) An older brother had fever blisters two weeks previously

    (E) Inoculation of HeLa cultures with vesicle fluid would have no visible effect

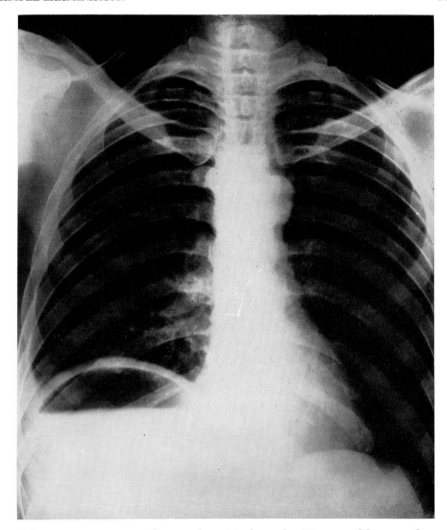

The roentgenogram shown above is that of a 50-year-old man who has had upper abdominal pain, fever and vomiting for three days.

4. This clinical picture is probably due to which of the following?

(A) Amebiasis
(B) Suppurative cholangitis
(C) Ruptured peptic ulcer
(D) Abdominal situs inversus
(E) Emphysematous cholecystitis

Questions 5–6

The following chart shows the influence of spironolactone on a 40-year-old man. Examination of the optic fundi showed arteriovenous nicking. Plasma volume was increased. Urinary excretion of 17-hydroxycorticoids (24-hour) was within normal limits.

The dotted horizontal lines on the urine sodium and urine potassium sections indicate the intake of these ions. "S.R." on the chart means secretion rate

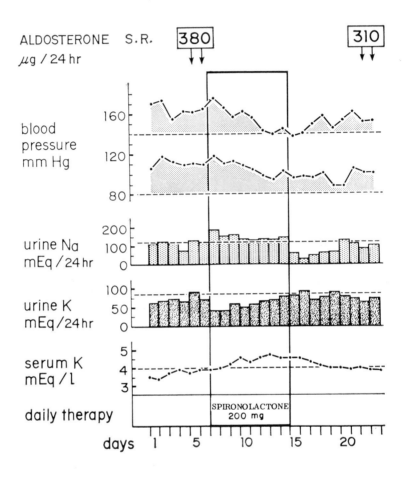

5. Which of the following is the most likely diagnosis?

    (A) Renal vascular hypertension with secondary aldosteronism
    (B) Malignant hypertension with secondary aldosteronism
    (C) Benign essential hypertension
    (D) Primary aldosteronism (Conn's syndrome)
    (E) None of the above

6. The most valuable single diagnostic procedure would be

    (A) renal biopsy
    (B) renal arteriogram
    (C) measurement of plasma renin activity
    (D) split renal function studies
    (E) none of the above

Questions 7–16
<u>Questions 7–16</u>

DIRECTIONS: Study the four electrocardiograms (A, B, C, D) shown on the following pages. For each numbered word or phrase below, select the answer in accordance with the following:

(A) if associated with the pattern shown in electrocardiogram A
(B) if associated with the pattern shown in electrocardiogram B
(C) if associated with the pattern shown in electrocardiogram C
(D) if associated with the pattern shown in electrocardiogram D
(E) if associated with none of the electrocardiographic patterns shown

7. Hyperthyroidism

8. Digitalis is the drug of choice

9. Hypokalemia

10. Hyperkalemia

11. Heart rate varies with respiration

12. History of paroxysmal tachycardia since childhood

13. Commonly found in children

14. Administration of anticoagulants may be of value

15. Digitalis toxicity

16. Paradoxical pulse

Study the four electrocardiograms shown below (A, B, C, D). Then answer Questions 7–16 on page 157.

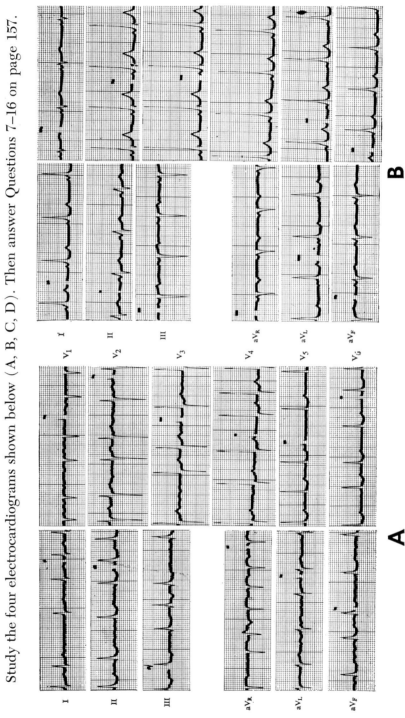

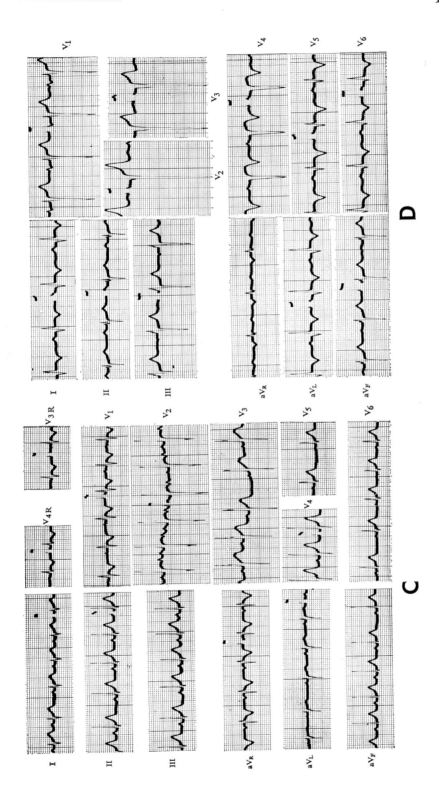

Questions 17–18

DIRECTIONS: The questions related to the pictorial material shown below are examples of the use of such material and item type X. Select each alternative that you think is right. All, some, or none of the alternatives may be right.

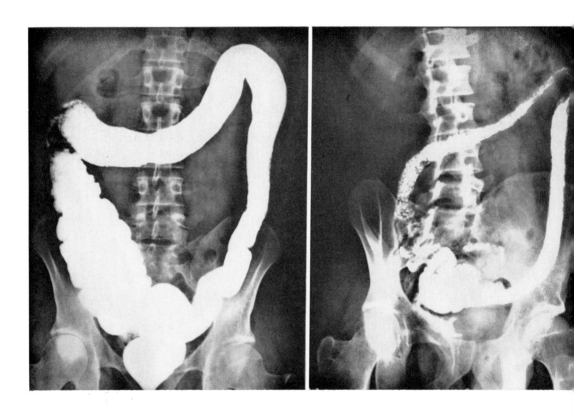

17. Which of the following might be expected in association with the roentgenographic findings shown above?

      (A) Arthritis
      (B) Megaloblastic anemia
      (C) High peaked T waves on electrocardiogram
      (D) Uveitis
      (E) Pulmonary cavitation

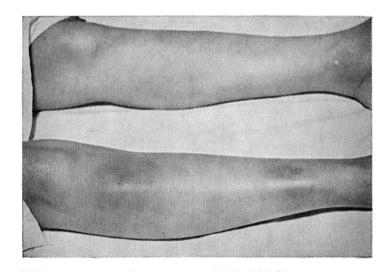

18. The lesions shown above are associated with

      (A) ulcerative colitis
      (B) tuberculosis
      (C) coccidioidomycosis
      (D) sarcoidosis
      (E) primary syphilis

Part III—Examples of Patient Management Problems (PMP): Questions 1–45

Name_____
    (Print)   Last   First   Middle

Candidate Number_____Examining Center_____

NATIONAL BOARD OF MEDICAL EXAMINERS

PART III—SECTION C

Time Allowance—3½ Hours

GENERAL INSTRUCTIONS

This is a test of your ability to manage patients. You will be given an opportunity to order diagnostic studies and procedures, to prescribe therapy, and to make decisions regarding each of a number of patients. Your task is to determine which procedures and therapeutic measures you consider appropriate, just as you would be expected to do if you were managing an actual patient.

A series of problems is associated with each patient. For example, the problems concerning Patient A are identified as Problem A-1, Problem A-2, Problem A-3, etc. The problems for each patient should be undertaken in the order in which they are presented.

Initial information is given for each patient in the printed test booklet. Following the initial information, the first of a series of problems (Problem A-1) for that patient (Patient A) is presented. Each problem consists of a numbered list of possible courses of action arranged in random order. You are not told how many courses of action are correct; for each problem, your task is to select those courses of action that you think should be done for this patient at this point in time, and to erase in the answer book the blue rectangle numbered to correspond with this choice. The response that appears under the erasure may lead you to select other procedures within the same problem, or you may decide to make other choices quite independent of information already obtained.

In general, the following kinds of responses will appear under the erasure for correct as well as for incorrect choices:

(1) When you order a diagnostic study (e.g. blood glucose, electrocardiogram, etc.), specific data will be reported.

(2) When you order a diagnostic procedure (e.g. liver biopsy, thoracentesis, etc.), specific data will be reported, or the response will indicate that the procedure was scheduled, done, or requested.

(3) When you order a therapeutic measure, the response will indicate that therapy was given, ordered, or started.

In the scoring of these problems, you will be given credit for correct choices; you will be penalized for errors of commission (selection of incorrect courses of action) and for errors of omission (failure to select correct courses of action). Any erasure which reveals any portion of the underlying answer will be treated as a total erasure. (Slight imperfections in the ink overlay will not be recorded as erasures.)

A sample problem is given on the back cover of this booklet. For practice purposes, you may proceed with this sample problem now.

Do not break seal until you are told to do so.

PATIENT A

There are 5 problems related to Patient A. These 5 problems should be undertaken in sequential order. Choices within each problem, however, may be made in any order.

General Information

A 45-year-old man is admitted to the hospital because of pain in his right hip and pelvis, especially when walking. He had lost 30 pounds in weight in the past year, during which time he did not feel strong or well enough to work. Three months prior to admission, he developed an acute upper respiratory infection and noted an increase in his symptoms with generalized "pain in my bones and stiffness of my joints." At that time, he also noted generalized numbness with tingling and stiffness of his hands; he had difficulty talking because his jaws and lips became stiff, making it difficult to form words.

Twenty years earlier he had had similar symptoms which he described as "pain all over." At that time, he was studied at a hospital for bone and joint disease, where he was told he had "osteoporosis." During the intervening years, he has been relatively well.

Physical Examination

Temperature is 37.0 C (98.6 F); pulse rate is 80 per minute and regular; blood pressure is 120/80 mm Hg. The patient is well developed and appears well nourished. The lungs are clear to percussion and auscultation. The heart is normal in size; there are no murmurs. The abdomen is protuberant but no masses or organs are palpable. There is pain in the right groin on palpation but no mass can be felt. There is 2+ edema of the legs but the extremities are otherwise normal. Neurological examination shows no abnormalities. Walking causes severe pain in the right hip and pelvis as well as pain in the feet.

Initial Laboratory Studies

Hemoglobin	10.0 gm/100 ml
Hematocrit	35 per cent
Leukocyte count	6,800/cu mm; polymorphonuclear neutrophils 60, lymphocytes 34, monocytes 5, eosinophils 1
Erythrocyte count	4,000,000/cu mm
Urine	Specific gravity 1.015, pH 5.5; protein 1+, sugar and acetone negative; microscopic examination: 3–4 WBC, 1–2 RBC per high-power field; no bacteria, casts or crystals
Roentgenogram of the chest	Lung fields clear

Problem A-1

With the understanding that all elements of the history are important, which of the following inquiries are specifically pertinent with regard to this patient's problem?

1. Appetite

2. Consumption of citrus fruits, juice, or foods containing ascorbic acid

3. Frequency, volume, consistency and description of stools

4. Transfusions, injections, "needles"

5. Exposure to people with cough, fever, or known infectious illness

6. Rickets in childhood, intake of vitamin D, exposure to sunlight

7. Sore throat, streptococcal infection, evidence or diagnosis of nephritis or kidney disease in childhood

8. History of hot, red, or swollen joints

9. Family history (siblings, parents) of skeletal deformity or "bone" pain

Problem A-2

You would now measure

10. serum transaminases

11. serum calcium and phosphorus

12. serum alkaline phosphatase

13. serum sodium, potassium, chloride, and bicarbonate

14. blood urea nitrogen

15. serum iron and total iron-binding capacity

16. serum acid phosphatase

17. phosphate clearance

18. antistreptolysin O titer

19. bromsulphalein excretion

20. serum uric acid

Problem A-3

On the basis of your findings up to the present time, which of the following studies would you expect to yield helpful information?

21. Intravenous pyelogram

22. Roentgenograms of the skeleton

23. Schilling (radioactive vitamin B_{12} excretion) test

24. Determination of fecal fat excretion

25. Glucose tolerance test (oral)

26. Determination of urinary methylmalonate excretion

27. d-Xylose tolerance test

28. Cystoscopy

29. Roentgenograms of the small intestine

30. Barium enema

Problem A-4

You would now order

31. liver biopsy

32. renal biopsy

33. bone marrow examination

34. biopsy of the small intestine

35. exploratory laparotomy

Problem A-5

Therapy would consist of

36. ferrous sulfate by mouth

37. transfusion with whole blood

38. vitamin D and calcium

39. a special diet

40. ammonium chloride

41. sodium citrate-citric acid mixture orally

42. parenteral injections of vitamin B_{12}

43. folic acid orally

44. ascorbic acid in large doses

45. exploration of the neck for parathyroid adenoma

PATIENT A
PROBLEM A–1

Patient A (continued)
PROBLEM A–2

Patient A (continued)
PROBLEM A–3

1. Normal appetite

2. Fresh orange juice daily

3. Greasy, bulky stools

4. None

5. No exposure

10. SGOT 30 units
SGPT 40 units

11. Calcium 4.6
phosphorus 1.8 mg/100 ml

12. 58 K.A. units
(normal 5–13)

13. Na 142, K 4.0, Cl 105,
HCO_3^- 27 mEq/l

14. 14 mg/100 ml

21. No abnormalities noted

22. Generalized demineralization;
bilateral pseudofractures of
upper femur and scapula

23. 6% excretion

24. 30 gm fat in 72 hours

25. Low flat curve

26. Normal

27. 1 gm of 25-gm dose excreted in 5 hours

28. No abnormalities seen

29. Dilated upper small bowel; segmentation and puddling

30. No abnormalities seen.

15. Serum iron 40, TIBC 380 micrograms/100 ml

16. 1.0 unit (K.A.)

17. 23 ml/min (normal 10 ± 5 ml/min)

18. 125 Todd units

19. 5% in 45 minutes

20. 6.0 mg/100 ml

6. No rickets, no exogenous vitamins; normal sun exposure

7. All negative

8. None

9. One sister has arthritis

Patient A (continued)
PROBLEM A–4

31. Moderate fatty infiltration

32. Normal

33. Erythroid hyperplasia. Absent iron stores

34. Flattened epithelial villi; round cell infiltration

Patient A (continued)
PROBLEM A–5

36. Ordered

37. Given

38. Given; serum calcium and phosphorus rise

39. Gluten-free diet given resulting in marked improvement

40. Given

41. Given

42. Ordered

43. Order noted

44. Ordered

45. Done

35. Patient refuses

Part I—Basic Science Answer Key

1.	D	26.	A	51.	B	76.	C
2.	C	27.	A	52.	D	77.	A
3.	A	28.	D	53.	E	78.	B
4.	B	29.	E	54.	A	79.	C
5.	D	30.	C	55.	D	80.	E
6.	B	31.	C	56.	A	81.	A
7.	D	32.	E	57.	C	82.	A
8.	C	33.	C	58.	E	83.	B
9.	D	34.	B	59.	D	84.	A
10.	C	35.	A	60.	A	85.	A
11.	C	36.	E	61.	B	86.	A
12.	B	37.	B	62.	A	87.	C
13.	A	38.	A	63.	E	88.	B
14.	B	39.	D	64.	B	89.	B
15.	D	40.	D	65.	A	90.	A
16.	C	41.	A	66.	E	91.	A
17.	C	42.	D	67.	A	92.	A
18.	D	43.	E	68.	B	93.	E
19.	E	44.	C	69.	D	94.	A
20.	E	45.	B	70.	A	95.	E
21.	D	46.	C	71.	E	96.	B
22.	D	47.	D	72.	D	97.	B
23.	A	48.	A	73.	A	98.	A
24.	D	49.	A	74.	B	99.	B
25.	D	50.	D	75.	C	100.	E

Part II—Clinical Science Answer Key

1.	E	26.	D	51.	C	76.	C
2.	A	27.	B	52.	E	77.	B
3.	D	28.	D	53.	D	78.	B
4.	A	29.	E	54.	B	79.	A
5.	D	30.	D	55.	E	80.	A
6.	D	31.	D	56.	D	81.	C
7.	A	32.	C	57.	C	82.	A
8.	A	33.	D	58.	A	83.	C
9.	C	34.	A	59.	B	84.	C
10.	B	35.	D	60.	D	85.	D
11.	A	36.	D	61.	E	86.	E
12.	B	37.	B	62.	B	87.	D
13.	C	38.	A	63.	A	88.	A
14.	C	39.	D	64.	B	89.	C
15.	B	40.	B	65.	D	90.	E
16.	E	41.	C	66.	A	91.	B
17.	A	42.	A	67.	B	92.	E
18.	D	43.	D	68.	A	93.	C
19.	D	44.	C	69.	C	94.	B
20.	B	45.	E	70.	E	95.	E
21.	B	46.	D	71.	C	96.	B
22.	A	47.	B	72.	A	97.	E
23.	A	48.	A	73.	B	98.	B
24.	B	49.	C	74.	D	99.	E
25.	B	50.	A	75.	A	100.	A

Part III—Pictorial Section Answer Key

1.	B	10.	E
2.	B	11.	C
3.	B	12.	B
4.	C	13.	C
5.	D	14.	D
6.	C	15.	E
7.	A	16.	E
8.	A	17.	A, D
9.	E	18.	A, B, C, D

Part III—PMP Answer Key

1.	Yes	25.	Yes
2.	No	26.	0
3.	Yes	27.	Yes
4.	No	28.	No
5.	No	29.	Yes
6.	Yes	30.	No
7.	Yes	31.	No
8.	Yes	32.	No
9.	Yes	33.	Yes
10.	No	34.	Yes
11.	Yes	35.	No
12.	Yes	36.	Yes
13.	Yes	37.	No
14.	Yes	38.	Yes
15.	Yes	39.	Yes
16.	No	40.	No
17.	Yes	41.	No
18.	No	42.	No
19.	No	43.	0
20.	No	44.	No
21.	No	45.	No
22.	Yes		
23.	Yes		
24.	Yes		

Index

175